R.M. PELUSO

Recovery of Smell & Taste

A GUIDE TO TRAINING & THERAPY

Ritual Communications
New York

Published by Ritual Communications

For information contact: Ritual Communications
www.ritualcommunications.com

Library of Congress Cataloging-in
Publication Data may be available.
ISBN: 978-0-9794674-8-6 (ebook)
ISBN: 978-0-9794674-9-3 (paperback)

Smell and taste are in fact but a single composite sense, whose laboratory is the mouth and its chimney the nose.

—Jean Anthelme Brillat-Savarin
(1755-1826)

The mind's capacity is limitless, and its manifestations are inexhaustible. Seeing forms with your eyes, hearing sounds with your ears, smelling odors with your nose, tasting flavors with your tongue, every movement or state is all your mind.

—*Bodhidharma*

CONTENTS

INTRODUCTION

How do you sense your world? Do you favor vision? Hearing? Touch? Smell? Or taste? Which is your greater pleasure, strolling through rose gardens or listening to music? There are those of us who prefer to smell those roses, even though we can't help but notice their vibrant colors. You may prefer the crunch of fall leaves underfoot to seeking out the scent of forests. But even the most visual or auditory among us will succumb to the right perfume. Because we aren't unisensory. Given a tantalizing cooking aroma, we are led by the nose, then the palate. Smell and taste. They matter. They impact us, however subtly. Hunger forces most of us to confront taste at least a few times a day. But like breathing, smell may be spectacularly overlooked. Until it's gone.

We didn't know much about smell or taste until the late 20th Century. What is smell? What is taste? What's the difference between taste and flavor, and why are these terms so often confused? What does it mean to never have smelled anything? To be born without that sense? Or to lose the ability to smell or taste? Once lost, can these senses be restored? This book explores such questions as it charts a return journey for some who have experienced loss, as well as those who would like to help loved ones and patients recover.

Smell used to be the step child of the senses, devalued and dismissed by scientists and philosophers. The novel coronavirus SARS-CoV-s2, or COVID-19, changed all that. Suddenly the word "anosmia" was everywhere, and no one was looking down their noses at olfaction anymore. Within the first couple months of the 2020 COVID outbreak in the United States, the loss of smell (anosmia) and taste (ageusia) emerged as early, sometimes solitary, symptoms. A month before the pandemic hit my New York City hometown, Italian doctors had been hearing pervasive complaints of sudden perceptual loss. Researchers scrambled. As a result, the crisis spurred investigations of these sensory deficits and the search for therapies.

It wasn't as if scientists hadn't been working all along on smell and taste, also called the "chemical senses." They had, but the research had been a mere trickle compared to a pandemic-inspired deluge. And smell and taste were not universally underappreciated. Always, they had been cherished by professional "noses" or tasters who toiled in the kitchens and labs of the food, beverage and scent industries, as well as those writing about such work. I should know, because I am one of them, a moonlighting food writer who began scribbling about chocolate while living her double life as a clinician.

Now semi-retired, I spent over 20 years as a Speech-Language Pathologist (SLP) before reviewing my first chocolate bar. During much of the pandemic, many of us food writers hunkered down in fear of losing livelihoods, to say nothing of our actual lives. More than that, we fended off the threat of losing the ability to perceive something indispensable to our very identities, our reason for living. Flavor!

When I think of the word *flavor*, it signifies so much more than its literal meaning. It is the difference between the uninterrupted beige of the ordinary and the spicy sparks of colorful intensity that infuse life with excitement and passion. It's falling in love. Even if it's just for a few morsel-filled moments.

Until I became aware of COVID's theft of smell, taste, and flavor, I never had cause to seriously think how devastating it could be to lose these senses. I've lived my life obsessed with flavor. Yet, ironically, I'd taken those gifts of perception for granted. The lack of smell or taste was beyond my imagination. But in 2020 such a possibility slowly worked its way into my consciousness. As I imagined existence without these senses, it became clear that loss meant hardship and disruption, not just for someone like me, but for anyone.

Getting to fully grasp the consequences of sensory deprivation took time. It would have been easier to let a self-protective curtain of denial descend. But that would solve nothing. Fear had to be confronted. So I prepared to wage my own personal war against COVID.

The first thing to do before going into battle is gather intelligence to understand the nature of the beast. Research. How did COVID attack? What were the best defense strategies? If the virus managed to break through and take out someone's smell or taste, how did that person recover? I wondered whether my odd blend of clinical and aesthetic backgrounds might be of some service. I engaged both my clinical and food-tasting skills to search for therapeutic possibilities as I immersed myself in the science of the pandemic and devoured anything written about smell, taste and flavor.

Flavor is, and was, essential for human evolution and civilization. But survival depends on taste and smell, the basic components of flavor. What happens if those perceptual abilities are suddenly gone? When impaired, their loss renders us helpless to detect a variety of dangers, from toxic foods to fire. We smell smoke or a gas leak. We taste the bitterness of poisons. A good sense of flavor tells us when something is subtly off, yet enough to make us sick.

The absence of smell, taste, or flavor impacts psyche and behavior. We may stop socializing because meals are tasteless or cooking aromas unpleasant. We may withdraw from loved ones because we no longer recognize their familiar odors. The shelter of home fails to comfort us without that whiff of lemony furniture polish or our beloved dogs still wet from the rain. Psychologically and emotionally, the lack of everyday odors, barely noticed as the backdrop of our lives, can suddenly send us spiraling down a hellish sensory vacuum. And when the loss is not complete, it can usher in a cacophony of distorted and distressing smells.

Perhaps, the worst part is the loneliness of struggling to find the words to communicate experiences that are often met with a shrug of incomprehension or doubt. Sensory perception is unique to the individual. It is a solitary experience. Even the sympathy of those close to us cannot overcome the barriers of each one's skin. And the skepticism of others can crush the spirit. Indifference marginalizes, intolerance alienates. The result— estrangement, withdrawal, depression, or anger.

For many, the pandemic made work and social interactions nearly impossible. At the height of the shutdowns, even the most extroverted had to turn inward to a degree. When there is disconnection, the stimulation of scent, taste, and flavor is a refuge that can open us to wider inner and external worlds. But for millions, the loss of smell and taste exacerbated the anxiety and depression in their shrinking existence, just when sensory enrichment was most needed.

As you will see, COVID isn't the only thief of smell and taste. These losses can be total or partial, permanent or transitory, congenital or acquired. Onset can be gradual, almost imperceptible, or shockingly sudden, the sequelae of other viruses, nasal polyps, sinus infections, allergies, head trauma, cancer, toxic exposure, or common medications. Anosmia (the inability to smell), hyposmia (weak smell perception) or dysosmia (distorted smell perception) can be the harbingers of tumors or neurologic diseases, such as Parkinson's or Alzheimer's. Chemical sensory impairments often present years in advance of other clinical symptoms. And diminution of smell and taste is common among the aged. Too often overlooked, weakened smell and taste contribute to decline in the elderly.

Perhaps the only silver lining to COVID is that it opened the flood gates for funding, research, and innovation that are likely to yield benefits for decades to come. But it has been at a gut-wrenching price. During the early days of the pandemic, everything was new, puzzling, and scary. Physicians didn't know much about this infection that was leaving a trail of death. In those first months of 2020, doctors had to follow the observations of clinicians thousands of miles away who were only a few weeks ahead. They raced to treat, to find answers, offering what they had, doing what they could, learning on their feet while stretched to the breaking point.

How quickly people forget those days as they rush to re-create a pre-2020 "normalcy" that is impossible to recapture. So a brief reminder. Because we owe it to those we lost not to forget. Whose family was not touched? Who did not lose a friend or acquaintance? We lost over a million Americans to COVID, and we're still not done. Over 30,000 died just this summer of 2022, while their neighbors ran around unmasked, believing it was all over. Infected heads of state and celebrities, staff shortages, cancelled air flights, and all manner of disruptions say otherwise.

Medicine is still struggling to understand COVID because it is complex, affecting so many systems of the body. Scientific investigation, traditionally slow, has been shaken from that pattern. Speed has been injected into the process. Studies that used to take 5 years from inception to publication now make it to pre-print online in 18 months or less. Sometimes this research is found to be flawed under peer review. But that's all a part of doing science in a pressure cooker.

In the beginning, there was a dearth of information for patients too. And to fill that void, self-help groups sprang up on social media. At the forefront was Christine Kelly, founder of the UK's *AbScent*, who lost her own sense of smell, first through an unspecified infection, then again from COVID. Another founder of a UK-based group, *Fifth Sense*, Duncan Boak lost his ability to smell in 2012 as a result of a head injury. Both founders independently networked with physicians, researchers and organizations, such as university-based smell and taste clinics on both sides of the Atlantic. They streamed video conferencing directly into the homes of participants who contributed important subjective observations and questions. Research findings, therapies, coping strategies and group support were shared over the internet. These forums became lifelines for many who found their ways to them.

Mid March 2020, as "lockdown" forced me from my clinical job, and food writing assignments were not enough to keep me occupied, I began reading whatever I could about COVID-19. I had become a subscriber to the Monell Chemical Senses Center's newsletters while working on my second tasting book. Now, a few years later, my inbox buzzed with bulletins from Monell and others. My clinical curiosity took the lead in pursuing links to information sources, but underlying that quest, a recurring question kept nattering at me. Could the way I approached professional tasting be of any assistance to people who couldn't smell or taste *anything*? And what could be done for patients who reported experiencing distorted or sickening aromas? What was going on there? Was therapy for sensory loss or distortion even possible? Any evidence in the research?

It turned out that sensory rehabilitation had already established a beachhead in Europe. Dr. Thomas Hummel of the

Smell and Taste Clinic at the Department of Otolaryngology, Technical University of Dresden Medical School had been investigating olfactory function and rehabilitation for years. Even before COVID, a small number of studies explored whether "smell training" was efficacious. The answer was moderately affirmative. Further investigations in the era of the pandemic began to support those initial findings. *AbScent* and *Fifth Sense* took inspiration from Hummel's work to promote smell training.

So, training might facilitate smell recovery and sensory healing. But who has been providing the instruction? Mostly otolaryngology (ENT) clinics associated with funded research groups. Training was pretty limited before online sources such as *AbScent* and *Fifth Sense* provided mass access. While these organizations remain important resources that help many, the course of training is left to the individuals to engage, or not, through technology. Participants in the online discussion groups lend support to those who might feel isolated or lost on their own. And while peer advice is often helpful, occasionally it's not well informed or applicable to another's experience. As anyone who's participated in support groups can tell you, a skilled moderator can make all the difference. *AbScent* and *Fifth Sense* do a pretty good job.

However, it is evident to me that smell training techniques also belong in a speech-language pathologist's toolkit. Here's the main difference between online training and therapy. An SLP has the background to keep up with the research broadly, and investigate narrowly, as patient needs dictate. Clinicians perform detailed assessments, formulate goals, measure results and evaluate outcomes, tweak the therapy to suit the individual, manage expectations, provide documentation, and interact with medical teams and insurance providers. That's vastly different from *training*.

My hope is that this book, through information and guided instruction, directly assists patients who suffer compromised chemical senses and those who provide support to those individuals. Also within these pages, speech-language pathologists will find techniques to incorporate into a therapeutic format. SLPs have specialized in chewing and swallowing (dysphagia) disorders since the 1980's. I count myself as a recipient of training by pioneers in the field, such as Justine Sheppard and Jeri Logemann. Logemann's work later touched upon the basic tastes and somatosensory effects. But there's still been little published on smell, taste and flavor with appropriate depth. The rehabilitation of the chemo-senses is a logical extension of what SLPs working in dysphagia already do. To facilitate an exploration of the subject, my colleagues are directed to the Appendix in this book, as well as the References section. General readers and patients may choose to skip those sections if they do not wish to wade through the science and references. The how-to aspects of smell and taste training in the first part of the book are presented in a reader-friendly, step by step format for people who just want to get better. But in the hands of skilled clinicians, part one becomes a manual for rehabilitation. My colleagues would do well to expand their scope of therapy practice to include people experiencing smell and taste disabilities.

ONE

TAKING IT PERSONALLY

But first, a quick digression for context and bona fides. Over many years, I had developed an interest in professional tasting, and after 2006, my hobby took on an increasingly serious turn as I became a contributor to a renown chocolate review website, the C-Spot.com. That experience, and my having developed a technique for highly focused tasting, led to writing a book in 2016 using what I called *Deep Tasting* skills to help others fully experience chocolate. About that same time, there was a lot of interest in pairing chocolate with other foods and beverages, so I began collecting data, resulting in a second book describing a system to pair chocolate with whiskey. Later, my database expanded to include cheese.

Being able to describe the characteristics of these three culinary treasures of the Western World and how to pair them led to publishing opportunities. In 2018, Whisky Magazine (UK) invited me to write a column on pairing chocolate, whiskey and cheese, and over the next couple years, I found myself writing for American Whiskey Magazine and Cheese Connoisseur Magazine. Those are some of my credentials as a skilled taster and food writer.

But decades before the food writing, the American Speech-Language-Hearing Association (ASHA) awarded me the Certificate of Clinical Competence after earning a masters degree from Columbia University. Not wanting to confuse patients or readers, I've always maintained separate professional tracks. So all my clinical credentials remained under my maiden name, and all my food-related publications carried my married name. Now that you might have an inkling of why I thought I could undertake the writing of this book, let's return to the pandemic which had just turned personal.

In the winter of 2019-20, we in New York began hearing about a horrible virus in China, then Italy, that was causing a high rate of deaths by pneumonia. COVID would prove to be more complicated than that, but those were the initial reports. And they were terrifying enough. I had just been assigned an article on truffle cheese by Cheese Connoisseur Magazine. In early February, I booked an interview and, with great trepidation, approached the showroom of an Italian truffle importer, tactfully asking my contact whether anyone at their showroom had arrived from Italy recently. Relieved to hear that no one had, I was able to conduct the interview.

As a practicing germaphobe who's been rehearsing for the next pandemic for years, much to the bewilderment of fellow riders, I had masked in the New York subways during every cold and flu season since the H1N1 Swine Flu pandemic of 2009. That was the one for which there had not yet been an available vaccine. My habitual precautions probably saved my life then and in 2020, because I masked while the COVID virus was stealthily infecting the city. It made no sense to me that health officials were telling us not to mask unless symptomatic. It was well known that a flu can shed virus a day or more before people know they're infectious. Therefore, it seemed prudent to err on the side of assuming asymptomatic airborne transmission was possible with COVID too.

Not only did the World Health Organization drop the ball by not declaring that COVID spread through airborne transmission, we also later learned that health officials in the USA had downplayed the need for masks as they were concerned about the public depleting a scandalously inadequate government stockpile of PPE (Personal Protective Equipment). The government was not prepared for a pandemic and had to reserve surgical masks and gowns for medical teams and first responders. But had officials been more forthcoming, and had everyone masked from the beginning, even with home made, multi-layer cloth coverings, we might have saved thousands of lives.

Instead, COVID was suddenly upon us. New York City became the American epicenter, and the city was too slow to take emergency measures. About the first week of March, a dear friend came down with COVID, losing her senses of smell and taste. While seriously ill with fever for 10 days, she thankfully did not develop the lower respiratory symptoms that led to so many hospitalizations and fatalities. But she was in her late 60s, and her health consumed me with worry as I witnessed the entire episode through daily check-ins via Facetime chats.

Let me describe the course of her illness. Being aware that COVID was around, she had been careful to follow the then current CDC guidelines in late February-early March, which tragically did not yet include the wearing of masks for asymptomatic people. We didn't realize how widespread this murderous virus already was in our own neighborhood. A couple weeks before New York went into the March 2020 lockdown, she said her nose felt congested. This was two days before developing a fever, so we were thinking she just had one of her many recurrent allergy attacks or sinus infections. Then she complained she could hardly smell or taste anything. I informally assessed her ability to smell and taste, discovering that she could detect sweet and salty, two of our five basic tastes. Her deficits seemed to be mostly smell, and by "taste" she actually meant the ability to experience flavor. People often confuse the two terms.

A quick explanation of the difference. There are basically only 5-basic tastes, sweet, sour, salty, bitter and umami (savory) picked up mostly by the tastebuds on the tongue. Flavor is complex, involving retronasal smell, which is experienced upon exhalation during chewing and swallowing as aromas travel up the oropharynx to the nasopharynx. These retronasal smells combine with the 5-basic tastes, plus the somatosensory inputs of pressure and light touch (texture), temperature and pain. Sensory information also comes from proprioception, which some propose as a 6th sense, but that discussion is beyond our purposes in this book. Vision and hearing affect the perception of flavor, too. Complicated, right? Here's the takeaway: Flavor is created in the brain through the integration of all these sensory inputs. I'll flesh out these processes in a little more detail later on. Back to my friend.

During her illness, my friend's deficit fluctuated on any given day, from no smell (anosmia) to weak (hyposmia) and distorted smells (parosmia). Unbeknownst to me at that moment, parosmia would turn out to be a good prognostic indicator that she might spontaneously recover. As she began battling ten days of fever, nausea and fatigue, she had to force herself to eat because things smelled so unappetizing. She ate as nutritionally as she could in the morning, before her afternoon fever set in. We tried to make good use of the time she wasn't sleeping, to talk her through breathing exercises, naively thinking we might prevent the dreaded respiratory effects of COVID. Fortunately, she never developed a serious cough or lung involvement. I have no idea whether the breathing exercises had any effect. It's likely she just had a milder case of the virus, nasty as it was. But in the face of insufficient information, you use whatever you can in the hope that it might be even remotely helpful.

For her hyposmia and parosmia, I recommended that she practice smelling familiar things she had in her home: cinnamon, oranges, apples, even coffee that was currently so aromatically displeasing. "See if you can smell more tomorrow. Keep a journal," I'd say to her at those times when she could hardly smell a thing. "As you take whiffs of the aromas, actively try to remember what they smell like. Use your imagination to fill in what's missing." Even though I had some basis for my recommendations, it felt like I was flying by the seat of my pants, as I coached, encouraged and cajoled.

Okay, the guidance wasn't entirely materializing out of thin air. I had a basic idea of sense memory from my work as a professional taster, and a rudimentary understanding of neurology from my training as a speech-language pathologist. But at that point, without any COVID-specific research, I was forced to improvise, and that meant relying on intuition to fill in.

My scientific knowledge of smell and taste was still primitive, with good reason. While I had learned much about hearing, vision, oral sensations, chewing, swallowing, breathing, phonation and speech production, as a student clinician, the science of smell and taste only gathered momentum after the discovery of olfactory receptor cells in 1991 by Linda B. Buck and Richard Axel. I learned a bit about smell and taste from my work as a food writer. But in-depth olfactory research, no. It was not a major area of focus for SLPs. I had taken a lot of postgraduate courses in swallowing disorders since 1991, but not a lot about smell and taste was discussed.

In order to be of any help to anyone else going forward, and to write this book, I had to close major learning gaps, such as, the latest on the anatomy and physiology of smell and taste, and COVID-specific and chemosensory loss in general. Then I had to research any evidence-based treatments. I had a lot of work to do. But during lockdown, I had the time and discipline to take on the challenge.

Meanwhile, you might like to know, that my friend recovered almost completely within two weeks from that first wave of Wuhan COVID. She was extremely lucky not to suffer any strokes, or heart or lung disease. She gradually overcame any fatigue, and her brief bouts of brain fog also disappeared within about a month. Every day, as I read postings from people suffering from Long COVID, I am shaken and viscerally reminded how fortunate she was in recovering so well. She has since taken all her vaccinations and boosters, wears masks in public indoor spaces, is careful about risk exposure, and has avoided reinfection. She has not taken her recovery for granted, and has not fallen for the popular delusion that COVID is over. Perhaps it will be by the time you read this. But it certainly isn't, as of this writing.

TWO

EVOLUTION THROUGH THE NOSE

I doubt that philosophers and scientists who have historically underestimated the human sense of smell ever shopped for a simple cantaloupe. Selecting the perfect melon starts as a visual event. We see it, we pick up it. Check that it isn't too green, no dents or cracks, no mold. Then, if you're like me, you put it to the ultimate test. You lower your nose to the green spot where the base of the stem once was, and you take a sniff. If it has a pronounced fruity aroma, you know from experience to expect that it's ripe, fleshy and sweet. You may shrug off the process as just something your mother taught you. But trust me, this is evolution at work, both biological and cultural.

Acceptable smells, tastes and flavors are encoded in our DNA, not just learned. And that which *is* learned starts earlier than you may think. Infants exposed to flavors in the womb show distinct preferences for those same ones after birth. They continue to acquire preferences and dislikes at the breast and in the highchair. Long before they can walk or talk, baby brains are like little sponges soaking up the aromatic preferences and biases of their culture.

But back to our cantaloupe. We haven't even put a morsel in our mouths, yet we call up aroma and flavor memories of the ideal melon in order to compare that to the fruit before us. This is a complex series of neurological processes that modern brain imaging technology, such as MRIs, among other investigative tools, are helping us to map out. Aroma is just one synapse away from the brain's olfactory bulb, the most direct route into the cerebral cortex of any of our 5 senses. Smell is represented by more specialized receptor cells than any other sense. In other words, we were built around our noses as surely as any of our canine companions, albeit our smell spectrum; that is, the detection and dynamic range, vary somewhat from theirs. Just because we cannot hear a dog whistle doesn't make human hearing poor. Mozart would beg to differ. And we are not inferior smellers. We are *different* smellers. Ancient philosophers and scientists who concluded that smell in the human species wasn't strong enough to merit much attention were dead wrong on that point.

When we *nose* that cantaloupe, we are one with all our hunter-gatherer ancestors who have passed wisdom down to the present generation. Smell, and our closely related sense of taste, enabled us to survive and to seek sustenance from plants and animals. If a melon doesn't smell ripe, our sensory intelligence figures it can give us a stomach ache. But that is the least of it. Humans learned to apply chemosensory perceptions and memories to all the foods to which they were exposed. We spat out the sour taste of spoilage, the bitterness of toxins. We built fires in order to destroy pathogens and release nutrients that weren't as readily available to us in their raw states, and by the same process, discovered that food could smell and taste better through applying heat.

Cooking enhanced aroma and flavor through a chemical process called the Maillard Reaction which occurs when high heat interacts with the amino acids in proteins. Anyone who has ever pan-browned meat is familiar with the tasty results. Minus the protein, the process is called caramelization. Cooks learned to caramelize onions and other vegetables, as well as to brown and roast spices, thus laying the foundations for the world's traditional cuisines. Families and communities gathered to share meals. As our ancestors pushed the flavor envelope by developing the tools and technologies to nourish their communities, they would later share foods through trade. Flavor drove culture and civilizations!

Our noses also protected us and helped propagate our species. Smoke on the wind meant to flee from a burning forest. The crisp, clean air that precedes snow warned us to take cover. The scent of people repulsed or attracted us, consciously, by suprathreshold levels of odors, and by those that are subthreshold or below consciousness, such as pheromones. Perhaps, we pick up chemical signals of aggression, illness, love, kindness, and many other states subconsciously. We may see why a person's manner seems trustworthy or is to be avoided, but we may also unconsciously smell why we "just have an intuition" about someone. Perhaps we are only a few research studies away from understanding the olfactory basis for some of our responses.

Smell, taste, and flavor were the bricks and mortar, or more accurately, the adobe, of culture. People point to the domestication of animals or agriculture as the beginnings of civilization. But to me, neuroscientist Gordon M. Shepherd was right to point to fire and flavor as the ultimate game-changers that preceded all that. Fire to warm ourselves, and to keep predatory animals at bay, to light our way, to create sacred rituals, later to smelt metal for weapons and jewelry, and to transform clay into food-containing pottery.

Flavor and fire traveled together, closely at first, then along less obvious parallel trajectories. No matter how far we have extended our fire-born technologies into the modern age, our quest for flavor has never stopped. When you think about developments that enabled humans to travel in space, food technologies went hand in hand with rocket boosters and computerization. People seldom think about the food. But astronauts could not consume rocket fuel or electronics! Essential nutrition in space required flavor on deck.

Without smell and taste, there is no perception of flavor. It is an impoverishment, a blow to the spirit, and a disability with severe consequences that must not be underestimated. When we experience an absent or diminished olfactory or gustatory sense, we need to know how it has come about, what the implications are, and how, if possible, to recover or rehabilitate them. Without smell and taste there is no flavor. And flavor is essential to our well being, our very lives, and our path to progress as a species.

THREE

SCOPE OF THE PROBLEM

In the Introduction, you read that COVID isn't the only cause of compromised smell and taste. It's just been the first to get so much attention. Chemosensory disabilities have always been with us, and will be long after COVID ceases to plague us. Pre-pandemic research by the Center for Disease Control and Prevention's (CDC) National Center for Health Statistics (NCHS), as reported by Hoffman et al. in 2016, found that in adults over age 40, 12.4% in their sample experienced olfactory dysfunction. That corresponded to 13.4 million in the general population in 2011-12, at the time of the survey. Smell loss increased with each decade of life until reaching 39.4% in people over the age of 80. Other studies of more homogeneous populations suggest the prevalence may be significantly higher, up to 80% in people over 75 years old, according to Brämerson et al. (2004) in Sweden, for example. Most alarming, according to the American NCHS study, among persons aged 70 and older, 20.3% were unable to identify the smell of smoke, and 31.3 %, natural gas. That means chemosensory loss is not just a matter of reduced quality of life; many elderly are forced to rely on electronic detection devices for safety.

We don't know how long the COVID pandemic will persist. Even with vaccination programs well underway in 2021, I thought that the coronavirus might linger at civilization's periphery, flaring up in small clusters from time to time. Since the Omicron variants arrived, that view now seems naive. Immunization didn't eradicate the virus as in the case of polio or small pox. The COVID vaccine didn't prevent the infection as effectively in the later variants as it did with the original Wuhan strain. Instead, the SARS-2 virus found a safe haven in which to mutate into more infectious forms among the immunocompromised, as well as in those unwilling or unable to take mitigation efforts, such as simple masking. As a result, we may never be entirely free of some version of COVID. For sure, we need updated vaccines that broadly target and anticipate mutated variants. These are supposedly, hopefully, arriving soon.

Misguided attempts to normalize our lives without taking the simplest steps to prevent COVID spread has led to increased risk for post acute health problems, such as blood clots, strokes, heart attacks, diabetes, brain disorders, opthamological, and all manner of vascular, multi-organ and immunological disorders. "Living with COVID" has not been a winning proposition other than for short term political and economic gains that abandon the most basic principles of public health. As reinfections predispose patients to complications and disabilities, it's a ticking time bomb for millions of individuals, their families, and ultimately society. Eventually, everyone will pay higher insurance premiums and taxes. We already see the inconvenience of staff shortages resulting from the absences of the acutely ill and the pre-mature retirement from the work force of longer-term disabled persons.

How many years into the future we will live with the casualties of COVID? Most patients have gradually recovered, but the fate of a sizable number has been more open-ended. As of this writing, many people are still suffering from Post-Acute COVID Syndrome (PACS) or so-called "Long COVID" since early 2020. Over two years. PACS is also sometimes spelled PASC for Post-Acute Sequelae of COVID-19. Both PACS and PASC refer to the same phenomena of complex, persistent symptoms which kick in after the acute phase of the infection; that is, at approximately 4 weeks.

At a congressional hearing on April 28, 2021, Drs. Francis Collins of the National Institute of Health (NIH) and John Brooks of the Center for Disease Control (CDC) testified that there were ongoing studies to follow those "Long Haulers" for at least two years. Collins and Brooks anticipated that millions of people would require future medical and specialty follow-up. As we attempt to pin down the numbers of people who may acquire Long COVID, we can already see that Collins and Brooks were correct. As of August 2022, according to the World Health Organization (WHO), there have been more than 588,757,628 known COVID infections worldwide. Approximately 6.5 million have died. In the United States alone, there have been more than 92,000,000 reported cases, and over a million deaths. That means, given the reported percentages of PACS in relation to those who've had COVID in the United States alone, from 4.5-27 million may have or had Long COVID. Why such a range?

The prevalence numbers for PACS are fluid at this point. We are always a year behind, producing data based on last year's variants. Therefore, prevalence estimates depend on the variant involved, vaccination status, and how the data is collected. Many studies define fully vaccinated as having had just the 2-shot primary immunization, others include boosters. While not an issue for total number of Long Haul patients, it is a challenge for comparative analysis. Another problem has been that many physicians have been slow to recognize, let alone report, PACS. In terms of stating the prevalence of PACS, that has become increasingly challenging given the undercounting of total cases of infection since rapid antigen home testing has become common. In the United States, the home tests are reported on a voluntary basis. Of course, those who had asymptomatic or mild COVID infections might not have tested at all or even informed a doctor.

Among the earlier variants, prevalence estimates were up to 30% approximately for the unvaccinated. Among the vaccinated who suffered breakthrough COVID infections, estimates went to 10% approximately. Later it was estimated that 1 in 12 persons infected who are up to date with boosters may still get PACS. The CDC further broke that down to 1 in 5 vaccinated under the age of 65, and 1 in 4 over 65. More recently, a large, controlled study in the Netherlands conducted by Ballering et al. (2022) reported 1 in 8 persons experienced post-acute symptoms. As it turned out, those vaccinated and up to date with boosters may have been only 15% less likely to acquire PACS.

Again, we need to look at the time frame and the variants. At least one United Kingdom study suggested that the Omicron

BA.1 produced less PACS overall, perhaps only 4-5 % compared to the Delta variant's 10.8% (Antonelli et al., 2022). However, we are several variants past BA.1, and as of this writing, BA.5 seems to be highly contagious and causing more serious respiratory symptoms. Therefore, it's possible that these later variants will explode the number of people living with PACS. No matter how you slice it, millions of people are suffering with Long COVID right now. Some patients are taking years to recover, and for a subset of patients, it remains to be seen how long it may take to overcome PACS, if they do at all. Despite the available antiviral treatments, and the reduced severity of infections and hospitalizations among the vaccinated and boosted, we are still losing thousands of lives every month. COVID went from being an infection among the general public to a health crisis among the unvaccinated, then to an invisible pandemic fueled by denial. How many victims will turn up with long- term disabilities due to PACS? Anyone's guess.

Hopefully, the study announced by Drs. Collins and Brooks to better understand Long COVID will improve the education of medical professionals and lead to treatment options. Patients who have been vaccinated and boosted undoubtedly fare better, experiencing far fewer hospitalizations and deaths. But any infection with COVID puts the patient at risk of PACS and chronic disease, surprisingly no matter how mild the symptoms. Severity of infection is no predictor of Long COVID. In fact, even those with asymptomatic infections can suffer Long COVID and require specialty medical treatment and rehabilitation. While there appears to be somewhat more women and older survivors acquiring PACS, many with

Long COVID are under 40 and were physically fit before they became infected. David Putrino and his team at Mount Sinai Hospital in New York City have encountered Long COVID frequently in athletes who pushed themselves to recover. Therefore, PACS is not an affliction limited to the elderly or those with pre-morbidities, as originally thought. This fact will come as a shock to those who champion a healthy life style and think good food, nutritional supplements and exercise will protect them from the COVID beast. Epidemiologists know better. Your best chance to avoid Long COVID is not to get infected at all. And that goes for avoiding smell and taste loss too, because they are frequently among the persistent symptoms of PACS. Therefore, to protect yourself from recurrent smell and taste loss, you need to protect yourself against infection. That means staying up to date with vaccinations and boosters, and masking when there's a viral surge in your region or when traveling.

How does Long COVID affect smell and taste? Disordered smell and/or taste can be early to resolve along with the acute stage of COVID, linger on with a variety of PACS symptoms, or remain the only symptoms of Long COVID. The Netherlands study by Ballering and associates found that between 90-150 days after diagnosis, 7.6% still reported anosmia or ageusia. A similar prevalence was noted by Boscolo-Rizzo and team (2022) who demonstrated that the process of recovering smell or taste can extend to 2 years or more. There had been some speculation that the early Omicron variants may have produced fewer cases of smell or taste dysfunction, but that remains unsubstantiated, and even if it ultimately proves to be true, the data may not extend to the BA.5 or later variants.

Here's an important takeaway. Even if you are someone who is healthy and in the prime of life, if you've been exposed to COVID, get tested. Check for the latest CDC or FDA guidance on type and timing of those tests. Get a diagnosis on the record and into your physician's chart. Proof of infection is essential, and not only to facilitate the timely acquisition of therapeutics. Lack of proof can lead to denial of coverage by insurance companies. While a new study by Klein et al. (2022) suggests a few key biomarkers, such as low cortisol, may predict who might develop Long COVID, it will be awhile until anyone is routinely tested. As of this writing, no one can say with certainty who may end up with PACS.

Long term intervention and rehabilitation are expensive, possibly open-ended time-wise, and you may be unable to work. According to the CDC, since July 2021, persons experiencing Long COVID can qualify as disabled under the ADA, the Americans with Disabilities Act. So, test or get tested whenever you suspect you might have been exposed, no matter how well you may feel presently. Document, document, document!

Wondering whether you have Long COVID? Here's a list published by the CDC of currently recognized, most commonly reported symptoms, as updated in July 2022.

<u>General symptoms</u>

- Tiredness or fatigue that interferes with daily life
- Symptoms that get worse after physical or mental effort (also known as "post-exertional malaise" or PEM)
- Fever

<u>Respiratory and heart symptoms</u>

- Difficulty breathing or shortness of breath
- Cough
- Chest pain
- Fast-beating or pounding heart (also known as heart palpitations)

<u>Neurological symptoms</u>

- Difficulty thinking or concentrating (sometimes referred to as "brain fog")
- Headache
- Sleep problems
- Dizziness when you stand up (lightheadedness)
- Pins-and-needles feelings
- ** Change in smell or taste **
- Depression or anxiety

<u>Digestive symptoms</u>

- Diarrhea
- Stomach pain

<u>Other symptoms</u>

- Joint or muscle pain
- Rash
- Changes in menstrual cycles

The CDC has a wealth of information and resources for Long COVID on their website. They warn that many symptoms can be difficult to describe or explain and that many lab tests can appear normal despite symptoms being present. Therefore, the CDC offers advice on how to prepare for a visit to a physician. For more information, go to:

https://www.cdc.gov/coronavirus/2019-ncov/long-term-effects/index.html

BEYOND COVID

The cause of anosmia and ageusia is clear with COVID and is often identifiable following a disease or trauma. But sometimes the cause of smell or taste loss may leave medical investigators scratching their heads. The truth is, we don't always know why someone loses their senses. But we should spare no effort to nail down a cause (etiology) and diagnosis. We need to urge people to pursue as complete an explanation as possible, if for no other reason than to prevent the tragedy of someone concluding that it is imaginary. When presented with a patient complaining of changes in smell or taste, a physician should not come to a conclusion before turning over every diagnostic stone. No one's complaint of sensory loss should be dismissed, even if the patient has known mental health problems. It's dangerous to miss possible early signs of a terminal illness that might be cured if caught in time.

Unless you're living with compromised sensory perception yourself, it can be difficult to understand or to sustain compassionate support. But families and friends must give the sufferer the benefit of the doubt and be fierce advocates for them. In the case of tumors, prompt action can save a life. Early diagnosis can mean all the difference in treatment outcomes. Knowing the cause of a sensory loss can determine whether any intervention might even be productive. And when intervention is possible, an accurate diagnosis can inform our choices.

Given the pre-pandemic prevalence of smell and taste disorders from multiple causes, we can project that millions of people in the future will experience the loss of chemosenses, whether transiently or permanently. COVID has opened the flood gates for research. Advancement is never worth the human toll of COVID, but progress is the legacy we owe to the memory of all who have lost their lives.

FOUR

TYPES OF SMELL AND TASTE LOSS

RECOVERY

DEFINITIONS

While we've already introduced a few terms used to describe the loss, or degrees of loss, of smell and taste, here is a concise list with definitions readers may encounter in this book and other literature on the topic.

Smell	**Taste**
Anosmia—the inability to smell	Ageusia—the inabiity to taste
Hyposmia—reduced smell perception	Hypogeusia—reduced taste perception
Parosmia—distorted odor perception	Dysgeusia—distorted taste perception
Phantosmia—perceiving smells that do not exist, an olfactory hallucination	Phantogeusia—a taste hallucination
Hyperosmia—superior or heightened smell	
Dysosmia— distorted smell perception, including parosmia and phantosmia	

PREGNANCY-RELATED DISORDERS OF SMELL AND TASTE

People who have never personally known the loss or distortion of smell and taste may have difficulty understanding the distress someone may be going through when experiencing these altered perceptions. But a sizable portion of at least the female population may have some insight due to familiarity with pregnancy-related parosmia and hyposmia. Two-thirds or more of all women experience parosmia in early pregnancy and/or hyposmia in late pregancy (Cameron, 2014). Taste too is often distorted. These parosmias, hyposmias and dysgeusias normally resolve after the birth of the baby. While some women report hyperosmia, or heightened smell perception, Cameron suggests that this likely means specific odors are more intense, and usually in an unpleasant way. Odors can be overwhelming, off- putting, and nauseating, and the culinary culprits are often the same foods, containing the same molecular compounds, that offend those suffering from virus-related parosmia. Some of the suggestions for desensitization in this book might help with parosmia in pregnancy.

A number of women in online discussions report that after struggling to overcome parosmia during and after COVID, they subsequently became pregnant, only to again experience smell dysfunction. Imagine how disconcerting that must be! Parosmia during pregnancy can be stressful and worrisome enough for any woman, but the prior experience with COVID can re-traumatize the patients when it recurs. Particularly when parosmia or dysgeusia have been symptoms of Long COVID and taken many months to resolve, the pregnant woman may fear that they will never recover. However, most report that their sense of smell does indeed improve postpartum. There is no reason not to do smell stimulation during and after pregnancy. It is a calming, centering process that can provide a few minutes of quality self-care. And for those who may be slow to recover postpartum, aroma stimulation, as described in the training and therapy chapter, can help them feel a degree of autonomy, as well as facilitate olfactory restoration.

CONGENITAL ANOSMIA

According to the National Institute of Health (NIH), approximately 1 in 10,000 people in American are born unable to smell anything. These are the congenital anosmics. The known causes of this sensory disability include malformation of the nose or neural pathways, and genetic mutations. Those born without smell may be unaware of their disability until it is pointed out to them. Some with congenital anosmia have made it well into adolescence and early adulthood before clearly understanding their situations. People without the ability to smell since birth have one clear psychological advantage over those who acquire anosmia later in life. The congenital anosmics have never known a different reality. They have learned to navigate their world through a different set of expectations and strategies. Congenital anosmics must use other senses, just as the blind learn to rely on touch and hearing, or the deaf on sight. One day DNA and transplant technologies may be able to assist those who wish to smell or taste. It's coming. But current therapies haven't much to offer them.

Understand that congential anosmia is rare, and pregnant women who are congenital anosmics are rarer still. With that caveat in mind, it has been reported by Cameron that one unique feature of pregnancy in women with congenital anosmia may be that they do not identify specific food stimuli as triggers to the nausea and vomiting typical of the first trimester. That may point to, in some cases, a role for aversive conditioning as underlying smell-triggered nausea and vomiting. In other words, if a woman in early pregnancy experiences nausea or vomiting at the time of consuming a specific food, she may become triggered by that specific smell for subsequent encounters. That does not by any means suggest that all nausea and vomiting in the first trimester is conditioned. Nausea and vomiting occur due to physiological changes. But it is possible that stimuli-specific smell reactions might become associated with vomiting if they occurred coincidentally, then further encounters with the odor may evoke nausea and/or vomiting. Still, why a would a woman stop getting triggered during a later stage of pregnancy?

Although we can learn a lot from congenital anosmics, this book is intended for those with *acquired* chemosensory loss. Earlier, I mentioned that in a study of normal adults over 70 years old with acquired anosmia or hyposmia, many were unable to identify smoke, and/or unable to detect natural gas. They face the same perils as congenital anosmics. Fortunately, these days we have smoke and carbon monoxide detectors, so fire and gas are not quite the threat they used to be. When it comes to food and drink, risk can be reduced by heeding expiration dates or looking for signs of spoilage. While not perfect, modern technologies and safety regulations have made the lives of persons with smell and taste disabilities, both congential and acquired, less perilous.

ACQUIRED LOSS

Anyone who was born with smell and taste perceptions but lost those abilities along the way is said to have *acquired* the condition. Common causes of acquired anosmia are viruses, nasal polyps, sinus infections, allergies, head trauma, cancer, post-surgical injury, radiation, toxic exposure, common medications, and aging. How many of us can pass 55 without increasing our risks? Not many. Prescription drugs and surviving into our later years go hand in hand. Acquired anosmia and ageusia can also signal the onset of degenerative neurologic disease; such as, Parkinson's, Alzheimers, and Multiple Sclerosis, sometimes as far as 5 years in advance of other clinical signs.

Support and intervention are essential for the newly anosmic or ageusic to prevent anxiety, depression or withdrawal. Those who have acquired chemosensory loss will need to recover, relearn, or adapt through compensatory strategies. The prognosis for recovery varies with the cause (etiology) and the particular ways these sensory disorders manifest in individuals.

RECOVERY

Spontaneous recovery occurs when a deficit is a symptom of an acute, temporary, or self-limiting disease, such as those arising from viruses, allergies, or mild injuries. In other words, these sensory losses often resolve along with, or soon after, the acute phase of infection or injury. But not always.

Smell and taste training has been shown to facilitate spontaneous recovery in some cases of inflammation and infection. When the infection or injury is of short duration; for example, a week or two, sensory training may not seem necessary as spontaneous recovery is likely. But that cannot be not guaranteed. And the longer the loss of sensory input endures, the more vulnerable the brain, memory, and neural pathways become to the possibility of lingering damage.

There is research evidence, including controlled studies, supporting the use of smell training to facilitate sensory recovery. Among the most recent, one by Altundag et al (2022) that specifically studied Long COVID patients, found that those using smell training for 9 months more than doubled their smell recovery compared to a control group that chose no intervention. Altundag's team used a Modified Olfactory Training procedure which will be discussed alongside Hummel's classic version in chapter seven of this book.

Stimulation through training increases the thickness of cortical tissue in key smell centers of the brain, whereas the opposite, a shrinkage of cortical tissue, is seen in stimulation-starved olfactory systems. Previously, many medical practitioners thought that there was poor prognosis for recovery if it had not occurred within 12 months, but Dr. Claire Hopkins, an ear, nose and throat specialist and researcher in the United Kingdom, says that loss need not be permanent, even in cases of long-standing deficits. To paraphrase her message in a recent presentation to *AbScent* (March 2022), recovery depends on the status of the stem cells in the nasal epithelium. As long as inflammation is eliminated or sufficiently reduced, stem cells can do their work of regenerating the other cells along the neural pathways, and sensory stimulation can eventually get through. Recovery is still possible, even well after a year.

Medical diagnosis and intervention can take a long time. We cannot afford to sit and wait when we can be doing something to limit long-term disability. Inflammation, when it exists, needs to be a target of medical intervention. Regardless of degree of inflammation, it's better to err on the side of stimulation without delay. In addition, it is psychologically empowering to give patients a daily intervention they can use. Systematically working toward a goal is important to overcoming feelings of helplessness and depression that are so detrimental to healing.

Detailed descriptions of smell and taste rehabilitation are addressed in later chapters. But briefly, smell and taste training can begin informally by using aromatic and taste stimuli readily available in the home: citrus fruits, scented soaps and creams, menthol cough drops, vanilla, mint tea, basil or rosemary, and spices, such as clove, cinnamon, or nutmeg. Select the ones you most appreciated in the past. Just start smelling them, right out of the jar, several times a day, and allow any memories associated with their aromas to surface.

A word of caution to parosmics. Coffee and chocolate may have been among your favorite aromas previously, but can be particularly offensive now. Getting to like them again can take time. You'll need to retrain yourself to tolerate them first. That goes for anything you may have enjoyed before you became parosmic but seem unapproachable now. Be patient. It's a process.

Unless nasty parosmic smells are so extreme that it makes you actually vomit, Christine Kelly advises her followers at *AbScent* to gently push through the unpleasantness. That makes sense from a physiological standpoint, as persistence may facilitate a degree of adaptation or desensitization to the offending odor. Desensitization should be approached slowly, building up frequent, tiny exposures until the unpleasant aroma or taste is first approachable, then tolerable.

Be determined about all sensory stimulation, even if for only a few moments at a time. Repeat often, at least a couple times a day. Keep a journal. Note any changes in your reactions on subsequent attempts. If spontaneous recovery doesn't occur within two weeks, a stepped-up, methodical approach to sensory stimulation can be found within these pages.

Meanwhile, it's advisable to seek medical help. Get a diagnosis and learn your treatment options. The smell and taste training and therapy in this book are not substitutes for a precise medical diagnosis and treatment. If COVID is still circulating in your community or in a place you have traveled, you should get tested. Get the medical attention you need without delay to take advantage of new therapies that are becoming available every day.

SURGICAL INTERVENTION

In cases where there is an obstruction, such as nasal polyps, surgery may be required. When it comes to head trauma, brain tumors, or cancer of the nose, mouth or throat, recovery depends on the location and extent of trauma, and the nature of the medical intervention. Damage due to the surgery, radiation, or chemotherapy can be so involved that smell or taste may recover only partially, or not at all.

About a third of all smell loss due to nasal polyps will be restored after removal, but many do not recover immediately. Chronic inflammation may remain a challenge that must be addressed for maximal recovery of function. The patient will need to work with the doctor to get the inflammation under control and to manage it over time, particularly when recurrent sources of irritation, such as allergies, are involved. Meanwhile, smell training or therapy should begin, even as inflammation is in the process of resolving, and continue until sensory perception is fully restored. By then, stimulation will naturally broaden out to include the many aromas and odors encountered in everyday living.

Head trauma and injury to essential organs or key sensory, associative, or memory centers of the brain have a guarded prognosis. But some improvement has been reported by Langdon et al (2018) using smell training. A glimmer of hope for loss due to some types of head injury has also just emerged in the experimental trials of insulin spray, although findings are still preliminary, and further research is needed. New treatment options are emerging all the time. Therefore, patients, advocates and their medical providers need to keep up to date on appropriate experimental trials. Express interest to your medical team and inquire about joining research studies.

Cancer may require conservative or extensive surgery, radiation and/or chemotherapy. Each aspect of treatment brings challenges to the prognosis for recovery. As important as our senses are, the priority of intervention must be to preserve life. That point must be clear, life first, smell and taste, second.

So much depends on the extent of surgery and radiation. If inflammation can subside, and if there's a possibility that stem cells remain anywhere in proximity to the affected areas, stimulation training or therapy can be tried. It's important that the patient or therapist is informed of the extent of the damage and the prognosis for healing of the affected areas.

Hope needs to be based on at least a modicum of reality. Unrealistic expectations can lead to frustration and depression. An attitude of "let's see" or "let's try," is helpful but must be carefully balanced against futility.

DEGENERATIVE NEUROLOGIC DISEASES

When it comes to degenerative, neurologic diseases, we can suggest to the patient or their caregivers that they try sensory stimulation in an attempt to slow the process of loss. Will it work? We should clearly state what we know and don't know, and that we need more studies to say whether it truly helps or not. Keep in mind that it's essential to do no harm, whether physical or emotional. Therefore, I advise SLPs and others to ask the patient's doctor first if they know of any reason that smell or taste training or therapy would be contraindicated or harmful.

We should try smell and taste therapy to see whether we can facilitate new neural connections during early recovery from acute illness, injury, and in post-surgical periods. But a degenerative disease is a different situation. And we need to be transparent. We must be honest about our intervention based on any research evidence that exists, and state plainly the limits of our knowledge. Even when we cannot produce evidence-based data, and the clinician cannot implement the intervention as a formal goal, we can informally introduce sensory training to the patient or their caregivers provided they fully understand that we don't know if it will actually help or not. It's important to manage expectations and prevent frustration or deep disappointment. Health care providers have to be guided by ethics. We cannot permit patients to waste time or avoid pursuing an evidence-based treatment elsewhere in favor of just *trying* smell or taste stimulation. Think of the stimulation as an addition to, not an instead of, in such instances.

STAGES OF LONG TERM RECOVERY

When recovery takes place over a longer period of time, as in the case of Post-Acute COVID-19 Syndrome (Long COVID), it may proceed in phases, but it's important to remember that everyone's recovery will be unique to them. Over several months, the lack of ability to smell anything (anosmia) might transition to a fluctuating ability to detect odors in an on-off manner, or to faintly perceive odors (hyposmia). Alternately, or subsequently, the recovering patient may report unpleasant or unappetizing odors (parosmia). These odors may be offensive, even disgusting; for example, a food might smell like a burned substance, ashes, garbage, sewage or excrement. These off-putting odors may provoke nutritional or social avoidance leading to weight loss or isolation. When disordered smell or taste is a symptom of Long COVID, there can be sudden set backs in progress due to stress or fatigue. Often sleep disorders or post-exertional malais (PEM) related to Long COVID can cause fluctuations in smell and taste.

Some people experience odor hallucinations (phantosmia). In other words, the smells aren't actually there at all outside the person's brain or, at least, there are no external stimuli detectable by anyone with normal smell perception. Phantosmia is internally generated within the patient. After COVID or a virus, phantosmia may be a sign of a type of recovery but may not lead entirely to the pre-morbid sensory perception that was normal for that person. At times, recovery must mean finding a new normal.

Phantosmia can also be a sign of incipient disease rather than a stage of recovery. If olfactory hallucinations occur when there's been no viral infection or any other identifiable cause of smell loss, the patient should see a neurologist as soon as possible. The neurologist will probably order a CT scan or MRI of the brain to rule out tumors or any other lesions.

Researchers hypothesize that parosmia and phantosmia point to recovery by somewhat different mechanisms, from attempts to create new neural connections in parosmia, to the disturbance of normal inhibitory functions at various levels of the olfactory pathway in phantosmia. Anosmia that gives way to hyposmia, an off-on breakthrough perception, or parosmia, can be a positive prognostic indicator that recovery is in progress. However, the time horizon for recovery can be unpredictable. Some see progress within a month, others within 4 months, some only after 6-8 months. A small but significant percentage of patients take longer than a year. So it's important to stick with the smell and taste stimulation therapy and not get discouraged. Sensory training demands persistence and must become a routine part of life, like any other type of physical training.

SUPPORT AND GUIDANCE

Those who acquire smell and/or taste deficits need understanding, compassion, patience and support from family, friends and health professionals. Online support can be found through reputable, science-based organizations, such as the *Fifth Sense* and *AbScent*. See the Resources section at the end of this book. It is advisable to approach other social media platforms with caution as they may be sources of misinformation. Even within the chat of reputable organizations, it is important to separate the subjective, anecdotal or speculative from the science-based comments. Some people can be alarmists or simply have experiences that are uniquely negative. Add that the personality of the person is unknown to you. They may be prone to exaggeration, superstitions, or prejudice. They may give you inappropriate or ill-informed advice. You don't know what motivates a person. Disinformation can be dangerous. Beware of recommendations that may put you off a proven course of evidence-based intervention in favor of unproved substances or procedures. We saw too much of that during COVID from individuals eager to profit from investments in pharmaceuticals, and crackpots peddling all sorts of drugs and supplements that had no peer-reviewed clinical studies to support their efficacies. Don't fall for pseudoscience. Go to the CDC or ECDC websites and search by key words to pull up peer-reviewed research articles. The leaders of *AbScent* and *Fifth Sense* are reliable, so if you participate in those forums, and have doubts about something you've read, ask the moderators.

Sensory loss can be emotionally traumatic and cause disruptions in various areas of life, including favorite activities and relationships. What if your favorite restaurants have specific smells that suddenly repel you? That will mean finding other places to go, making alternative plans. Routines may need to change. Can you imagine how destructive it might be to find your partner's odor so repulsive that you want to avoid any form of intimacy? The scents a partner uses in their personal care may also suddenly offend. It's not the fault of either party, but less offensive products might have to be substituted. In order for a relationship to survive, a great deal of understanding, non-defensive communication, and co-operation in problem solving will be required.

Beyond mental and psychological impacts, support can make a difference to physical health, as it can be challenging to maintain weight and meet nutritional needs when the smell and taste of food is off-putting, even nauseating. A partner or caregiver needs to be flexible. Not only may they have to change the foods they buy, if any offends to a severe degree, they may need to cook at a time when the patient is out of nose-range.

TENDER, LOVING SELF-CARE

People with smell and taste deficits are advised to be patient with themselves in anticipating progress. They need to be diligent in self-care. It's important to remain realistic yet hopeful while working consistently with training, therapy and interventions. Sensory work needs to become as automatic a part of a daily routine as brushing teeth. Carving out a regular schedule for sensory training helps us to remember to do it. Make it a special time for yourself. It can be centering and emotionally grounding to devote sensory training sessions as a time for self-care.

PREVENTION OF SMELL AND TASTE LOSS

When it comes to aging, there are things you can do to protect those delicate smell and taste receptors of the nose and mouth, such as not drinking alcohol to excess. Studies have shown that low income people who live in areas where there is excessive air or water pollution present a greater incidence of smell and taste loss. Therefore, in addition to losing receptor cells due to natural aging, there are environmental threats to smell and taste. There isn't much you can do if you must live in such circumstances, but air purifiers, water filtration systems, and house plants might be considered.

The receptor cells in the nose replicate themselves every 3-4 weeks, while those in the mouth and tastebuds take 1-2 weeks to turnover. Nasal olfactory cells and tastebuds require time to regenerate. We've probably all had the experience of scalding our mouths on hot coffee. We usually recover within a week, if the injury is mild. But imagine ongoing injury that is never given a chance to heal and has long term effects. Therefore, be careful about daily alcohol consumption, smoking, or exposure to any caustic or chemical substances.

Many common medications cause dry mouth (xerostomia). We need to stimulate saliva production to moisturize the tongue and oropharynx in order to break down the molecular compounds in foods for uptake by oral taste receptors and the retronasal aromatic pathway. Both contribute to the perception of flavor.

For dry mouth, sip some water before consuming anything. Saliva is 99% water, but it also contains digestive enzymes and other important substances. There's nothing like the real thing. Therefore, if saliva can be stimulated, that is the best option. Other than medications, how can we produce more saliva? First, it's important to keep hydrated and your electrolytes in healthy balance. Also, before eating, stroking for a few moments on the lateral side of the tongue, half way back, with a spoon, raw carrot, celery stick, or lollipop, can stimulate saliva. Alternatively, try chewing gum or briefly sucking a hard candy. Don't bite it, and no need to swallow it. If you wish to avoid sweets, try a sugarless hard candy or chewing gum for a few minutes. Avoid glycerin swabs, however, because they tend to dry the tongue over time. Once you put the actual food of your meal in your mouth, slow down and chew longer to produce more moisture. Try the suggestions just offered. See whether these moisture- stimulating strategies create not only more saliva, but also more flavor for you.

If none of the suggestions above work, there are medications to reduce xerostomia. Discuss such options with a Primary Care Physician (PCP) or an Otolaryngologist (ENT).

AVOID SMELL RECEPTOR AND TASTEBUD FATIGUE

Being curious and trying new foods helps us pay attention to sensory stimulation and leads to better nutrition and flavor experiences. Variety is key. Tastebud and smell receptor fatigue happen when we consume or smell more than a few bites of the same food or drink in a short period of time or inhale the same odor repeatedly. For optimal flavor perception, we need to avoid sensory fatigue, also called habituation or desensitization. Therefore, eat more than one food at any meal and alternate among those foods frequently. Take water sips between bites. Taking more time to savor and enjoy each food is a helpful habit to acquire.

If you've ever shopped for perfume, you will probably be familiar with the desensitization that happens after smelling scent after scent without resting. Suddenly every aroma becomes muddled. Some perfume counters offer coffee beans to sniff as a way to "reset" the nose. It gives you a chance to rest the olfactory receptors that are sensitive to a particular set of molecules while engaging other receptors with the coffee beans. The smell and taste exercises you will find in this book can help keep your sense perceptions sharp.

FIVE
MEDICAL INTERVENTION

Let's suppose you've had a loss of smell and/or taste for more than 24 hours. Assuming the world hasn't changed by the time this book is published, even if you have a history of allergies or sinus problems, regardless of whether you've been vaccinated, you need to immediately rule out COVID-19. Call your doctor. Get tested!

At this writing, rapid home tests are available at pharmacies. Professional laboratory-affiliated sites may still be located in communities across the country offering PCR testing. Regardless of how or where you test, remember that you will need to provide documentation for insurance reimbursement, Medicare and Medicaid. A home test may not suffice. The more complications and treatment any disease presents, the more rock- solid documentation is necessary. If you can't find a test or testing service, ask your medical provider for guidance. A doctor's on-the-record diagnosis will be important to support your claim of infection. Whether from a virus or any other cause, beyond the duration of acute infection, if you have a persistent sensory loss, you should contact your medical provider and inquire about getting an evaluation.

A medical assessment for sensory loss begins with a Primary Care Physician or an Otolaryngologist; that is, an Ear, Nose and Throat (ENT) specialist. I'd see an ENT as soon as possible. Not to disparage general practitioners, but they have many diseases to worry about, including those of their subspecialties that may be unrelated to chemosensory loss. An ENT is more likely to have the instrumentation and sensory tests to provide a thorough assessment.

The evaluation process should include taking a thorough history of smell and taste function, as well as a description of the onset of the current sensory loss. That's where your recollections come in. Make note of when the symptoms started and jot down any descriptions you can.

At the ENT's office, the nasal passages will probably be examined with a flexible endoscope. Also, although still not frequently offered, it's highly recommended that a baseline description is obtained of how well you can detect, identify, and discriminate odors as measured by a standardized smell test, such as the Sniffin' Sticks or the UPSIT. These tests, discussed in this book's Resources section, are helpful in differentiating the patient's subjective impressions from an objective and quantified description of an olfactory or gustatory disability. People are often inaccurate in recognizing their loss or its magnitude. Retesting months later is useful in measuring recovery progress. The physician may also refer you for additional tests, such as a CT scan or MRI.

On the next page is a chart with an overview of some current diagnostic and treatment options that may be used or prescribed when patients with smell and/or taste loss present themselves for medical assessment. As mentioned earlier, COVID-19 has stimulated intense research and cross-disciplinary cooperation. We can anticipate more diagnostic and treatment options to become available. Due to the COVID pandemic, intervention is becoming more available locally, even for non-COVID causes of sensory loss. There are a number of smell and taste clinics included in the Resources section of this book.

Since smell training benefits patients experiencing a diverse number of diagnoses, err on the side of being proactive. Start sensory stimulation informally as soon as possible while waiting to see a physician. Progress with smell training can be slow, so be patient and stick with it.

EXAMPLES OF DIAGNOSIS AND TREATMENT FOR OLFACTORY LOSS

Onset Type	Diagnosis	Treatment
—No memory of onset	>Congenital	>None or Experimental
—Sudden onset	>Post infection	>Zinc Gluconate*
		> Smell Training
		> Supplements*
		>Pea-Lut **
	>Post traumatic	>Insulin (experimental)
		> Smell Training
—Gradual onset	>Aging	>Smell Training/ Compensatory
non-fluctuating	>Neurodegenerative	>Smell Training & Experimental Medication
fluctuating	>Post traumatic	>Smell Training
	>Idiopathic	>Smell Training

Testing & Procedures	Diagnosis	Treatment
—ENT> Nasal endoscopy	>Pathology:	
	-chronic allergic rhinitis	>Steroids
	-sinusitis	>Antibiotics/steroids
	-injury	>Surgery/other
	-polyps	>Surgery
—Standardized olfactory testing	>Description of perceptual loss, discrimination and identification ; Sniffin' Sticks, UPSIT, (see Testing)	
—Imaging >CT/MRI	>Volume of olfactory bulb/olfactory clefts	
>fMRI	>Dynamic function of cortical pathways	
>EEG	>Evoked potentials of olfactory centers of the brain	

*Anecdotal or insufficient data: : Alpha Lipoic Acid, Omega 3, Vitamin A drops-topical/nasal Herbal: Toki-Shakuyakura-San

**Pea-Lut (Palmitoylethanolamide and Luteolin) oral supplement demonstrated improved results for smell therapy in at least one study (Di Stadio et al. 2022).

Promising pilot studies:

—PRP Plasma, delivered locally by lavage, to promote tissue repair/ anti-inflammatory

—Basal stem cell transplant]

(updated from: Boesveldt et al 2017; Malaty & Malaty 2013)

GETTING THE RIGHT KIND OF MEDICAL HELP

If you don't live near a smell and taste clinic, consider contacting one for a referral to a specialist in anosmia and ageusia in your area. Since many of the clinics are associated with university medical training centers, their lists of providers are likely to include physicians who are most current with recent developments and able to refer patients for clinical trials. Check the Resources section of this book for a partial list of international medical centers and practitioners.

Evidence has been accruing against the effectiveness of over-the-counter and common prescription nasal sprays for reaching the depth of the nasal passages into the clefts where inflammation contributes to impaired smell. Method of delivery is as critical as the medicinal spray or rinse formulation. Several ENT sources specify that the patient must be positioned optimally; for example, lying on their side with their chin pointed up toward the ceiling. If you consider how most of us use nasal sprays, it becomes immediately apparent why we aren't getting up far enough to reach the right places.

The earlier the intervention the better. A small MRI study by Eliezer and associates (2020) demonstrated that obstruction of the Olfactory Cleft(s) was the location of the area affected by COVID-19, not the Olfactory Bulb. In that study, conducted at only a month post acute infection, smell loss appeared related to inflammatory processes still in the nasal epithelium and not in the brain. However, a more recent, much larger Oxford study by Douaud, et al.(2021), found otherwise. The Oxford study included hundreds of subjects who had been previously scanned, then seen post-infection, along with healthy control subjects. The authors of the study didn't mention how long post infection the patients underwent MRIs, but it was clearly longer than a month. They found a loss of gray matter in the cortical limbic areas that directly implicated the primary olfactory and gustatory systems. In other words, this suggests that shrinkage is the result of pathways starved of stimulation. The value of the Eliezer team study seems to be that it demonstrated, in patients who had not recovered their sense of smell within a month of onset, obstruction of the Olfactory Cleft(s) could still clearly be seen in the MRIs. The data from the imaging suggested a loss of smell, in patients with COVID-19, was related to a transient edema of the olfactory clefts, at least early on. Treatment implications point to the efficacy of the early use of steroid treatment, delivered by nasal irrigation to the Olfactory Cleft(s).

Could very early use prevent damage spreading to the olfactory centers of the brain and beyond? That remains to be studied. However, it has been suspected that the entry point for a virus to the central nervous system is the olfactory mucosa, and that is not limited to COVID. Independent of smell and taste specifically, studies point to general brain damage in Long COVID that manifests as "brain fog," memory deficits and impaired executive functions involved in organization and decision making. But just from the perceptual standpoint, a goal should be to minimize the shrinkage of the brain tissue related to the olfactory centers and pathways caused by the lack of sensory stimulation. Therefore, proactively reducing obstruction so that stimuli can reach the brain seems a compelling goal for intervention. As obstruction can fluctuate even before total resolution, sensory training or therapy of smell and taste should begin immediately to take advantage of every opportunity for stimulation necessary to preserve and rebuild neural connections.

EVOLVING REHABILITATION FOR POST ACUTE COVID-19 SYNDROME

David Putrino, P.T. Ph.D., is director of The Rehabilitation Innovation program for the Mount Sinai Health System and Assistant Professor at Mount Sinai's Icahn School of Medicine, as well as head of Putrino Labs in New York, NY. Dr. Putrino is a physical therapist with a doctorate in neuroscience and a specialist in computational neuroscience. He has worked with COVID patients since the early days of the pandemic in New York City. Mount Sinai was the first medical system in America to establish a program for treating Long COVID at their Center for Post-Acute COVID Care. Readers can view several Youtube videos featuring Putrino describing his approach and insights. One takeaway from his narratives is the potential for exertion and stress to cause flare-ups. This phenomena is now well known as PEM or Post-exertional Malais. Patients even slightly pushing beyond their limits pay a big price 24-48 hours later in terms of a resurgence of fatigue and other debilitating symptoms.

Putrino began to see similarities between Long COVID and dysautonomia, or autonomic dysfunction, that affects many organs, including the heart, bladder, gastrointestinal tract, pupils, sweat glands and blood vessels. Symptoms include those often described by patients suffering from Long COVID, such as brain fog, dizziness, blurry or double vision, exercise intolerance, swallowing issues, low blood pressure and orthostatic hypotension, syncope, sleep disturbances, weakness, and fatigue. Putrino's experience dispels the notion that healthy individuals don't suffer severe COVID or its aftermath. His patients, many young people in the prime of life and former athletes, most in their 20's-late 40's, reported feeling almost totally done in by COVID and Long COVID. They were not the elderly or infirmed. Most had COVID that resolved at home and were not critical enough to be hospitalized. We now know that severity of the acute infection does not predict the potential for being impacted by Long COVID. You can have mild or asymptomatic COVID and end up with PACS.

While I have not heard Dr. Putrino specifically address smell and taste issues, the loss and dysfunction of the chemical senses are very much a part of the Post-Acute COVID Syndrome experience for many. Stressors such as anxiety, depression, lack of sleep, other health issues, as well as exertion, can cause fluctuations in recovering smell and taste. As patients, caregivers, and clinicians, our takeaway from Dr. Putrino's insights is that we need to avoid flare-ups of smell and taste dysfunction through the careful calibration of activities and moderating of stress. Expectations of full normalcy leads to over-extending oneself which causes crushing regression and disappointment. Therefore, patients may need to accept a new normal, at least for the duration of PACS.

Life is challenging and does not always make it easy to practice good self-care. But for people recovering from anosmia and ageusia, managing sleep, stress, nutrition, and exertion must be part of the prescription. When smell and taste are the only residual long-term dysfunctions, it can be difficult for those around you to understand that "just getting on with your life," full speed ahead, and trying to get back to the way you were pre-COVID, can cause counterproductive set backs. Patients themselves can be so anxious to return to pre-pandemic normalcy that they may overlook the fact that what remains is really not normal, and that they have to find a new normal until they are no longer vulnerable. And the truth is, we don't know how long a person can remain fragile in some unseen way. People may seem to "recover" in a year, or two years. They may go back to work, fully engage with family and social activities, but we don't know what impact any other illness or emotional trauma may have. Can someone who seems fully recovered possibly experience a regression three years later? We simply don't have the data to answer that question yet.

We don't know what awaits the post-COVID patient a decade or two later, what time alone may trigger. Some viruses lie dormant and may suddenly wake up in a season pre-scheduled in their, or our, DNA. Think of varicella, childhood chicken pox, emerging as shingles in an 80 year old. Viruses are that unpredictable. Researchers recently found that for some people Epstein-Barr can be one of those dormant diseases that suddenly manifests many years later as Multiple Sclerosis. We are probably on the cusp of discovering a multitude of degenerative illnesses that could have entered the body as a simple virus.

It is currently underappreciated that it is important to avoid COVID infection. People mistakenly think it's like a flu or cold and getting it is to "get it over with." There's no evidence of enduring immunity. Such people fail to appreciate that they can get reinfected in a matter of weeks, and as each infection impacts the immune system, reinfections can cause more serious outcomes in the acute stage, post-acute state, or possibly lie dormant for decades. There's emerging evidence that reinfection increases risks for long-term debilitating conditions, such as PACS. Even mild and asymptomatic infections can set patients up for strokes, heart attacks, and blood clotting six months or a year later.

COVID is not the only virus capable of causing a loss of smell or taste. It's just been so recent, present and disruptive in our lives. If that wasn't the case, it's doubtful this book would have been written. But regardless of the source of your acquired sensory loss, there is material offered here that may assist you in recovering, help you to cope or compensate. The next chapters are hands-on practical, about testing for loss, stimulating and training our senses, and providing therapeutic tools for clinicians.

SIX
TESTING IS ESSENTIAL!

If you brew morning coffee only to find that you suddenly cannot smell it, or that the aroma resembles sewage, you should call your doctor. You likely have anosmia or parosmia, and you need to know why. But what if the onset of your sensory loss was so gradual that you didn't notice it? The aroma is just a little weak. That delightful jolt of java is increasingly, but subtly, unsatisfying. You're not sure what's going on. But you aren't alarmed, and it doesn't seem like an issue you need to take to a doctor. You think, maybe the beans are old. Maybe something's wrong with your usual brand. You try a new one, or switch to espresso. You brew it stronger. Then you notice feeling nervous. Of course you are! Because you're consuming too much caffeine. How can that be possible? You didn't even taste it!

What if your favorite dishes suddenly tasted flat? Most likely, your first instinct is to think, hmm…not enough salt. So you grab the shaker. Repeatedly. Then you pay a routine visit to your doctor and find your blood pressure's sky high. Unfortunately, too many people in the quest for flavor add sodium to the detriment of blood pressure stability. These scenarios are all too common.

The problem isn't old coffee beans or flavorless food, it's our old noses and the failure to detect moderate seasoning. There are ways to compensate. You can add herbs and spices instead of salt. You can brew your coffee stronger but reduce the amount you drink to prevent the overconsumption of caffeine. These are just a couple suggestions. You'll find many more ways to compensate for absent, weak, distorted or unpleasant flavors later in this book.

Smell and taste incrementally decline in normal people after age 40. The 2013- 2014 National Health and Nutrition Examination Survey (NHANES) investigated, in addition to the sense of smell, the intactness of bitter and salty taste perception. In the NHANES sample population, among subjects over the age of 40, with a mean age of 57.5, impairments of smell were found in 13.5%, and in 17.3% for taste. Overall, approximately 28.6% of US population had either or both impairments. Prevalence increased to 37.2% in men and 25.2% in women over 70. In persons over 80, the numbers exceeded 40%. That's a lot of sensory impoverishment! And the statistics are worse for minorities and the poor who are more likely to suffer risks to their chemosenses due to environmental and underlying health conditions. Deficits in smell and taste are more common than most of us think, yet before COVID-19, doctors seldom asked about sensory loss during annual physicals, not even of their elderly patients. How many primary care physicians ask today?

SELF-REPORTING

When sensory loss is dramatic or sudden, people will remark upon it to close associates or doctors, or report it when interviewed by researchers. But when it's gradual, quality of life slowly and silently slips away. When comparing reported versus measured (actual) loss, it is clear that the majority of those with gradually diminishing chemosensory perception tend not to notice their deficits or seek treatment for them. Nevertheless, these impairments can have serious implications for nutrition and health, both physical and mental. When a person eats less, or tries to compensate by using too much salt or sugar, that can have physical consequences such as weight loss or gain, and blood pressure or glucose spikes. In terms of mental health, it is easy to become depressed by the cumulative lack of pleasure when foods lack excitement. Such feelings are particularly true for more socially isolated individuals. Unfortunately, many elderly fall into that category. Increasing sensory stimulation can be one tool to mitigate depressing aspects of isolation.

It's easy to see the importance of assessing smell and taste in yearly physicals and wellness checkups, yet our senses remain woefully neglected in routine annuals. Even when the pandemic is finally over, healthcare providers would be well advised to ask all patients whether they have experienced any changes in the way things smell or taste in the last 12 months.

In addition, I'd advise health care providers to ask people over 50 the following:

- Think back to when you were approximately age 25. How would you characterize any changes in the smell or flavor of favorite foods?
- Are you eating or drinking less these days?
- Any change in your level of enjoyment of favorite foods?
- Do you find yourself adding more salt or sugar to your foods than you used to do?
- Are you substituting unhealthy foods, such as salty or sugary snacks, to compensate for a lack of satisfaction in your meals?

Healthcare providers can also use this opportunity to screen for chewing and swallowing issues which increase with age. Chewing can become problematic with the loss of dentition. Both chewing and swallowing can be compromised by dryness of the mouth, a side effect of many common medications. Readers can check on whether their medications cause dry mouth by asking a pharmacist, checking the drug prescription insert, or searching the Physicians' Desk Reference (PDR) online at https://www.pdr.net, or the consumer version, https://www.drugs.com. Without sufficient moisture, food residue can get stuck between the teeth or dentures and inner cheek or gums. Tongue movements sweep this residue away so that it can be swallowed, but that process can be a challenge with reduced moisture.

In addition, as we age, neural degeneration can mean it takes longer to trigger the swallow reflex, or to clear food from the back of the throat as it heads into the esophagus. This can lead to choking or aspiration. Aspiration occurs when food or fluid "goes down the wrong pipe;" that is, down through the vocal folds of the larynx into the trachea en route to the lungs, instead of down the esophagus en route to the stomach. When the elderly are otherwise healthy, mobile, with good respiration and have a strong cough, rare aspiration can be overcome. But lacking any of those strengths, aspiration can lead to pneumonia.

Sometimes there is a problem in the esophagus. The time it takes to clear food or liquid from the esophagus can increase due to reduced peristalsis. Chunks of meat or bread may feel stuck or painful. Also, it's possible that the upper esophageal sphincter leaks, so that fluids back up and can enter the laryngeal area. This regurgitation is what is meant by the term "reflux." Telltale signs include burning sensations, foul breath, and a nasty taste. Reflux sends corrosive stomach acids upward which is suspected of contributing to esophageal cancer. This seepage can also cause coughing fits that sometimes wake people out of a deep sleep. Again, in medically fragile people this can be a risk for aspiration pneumonia. Disorders of the esophagus need to be discussed with the primary care physician to rule out impaired peristalsis and reflux.

Health providers should ask:

- Does the patient find themselves coughing more frequently when they eat or drink? If so, how often does this happen?
- Does the patient ever wake up choking on their own saliva or reflux?

- Have they ever choked on a food and required assistance? How many times has this happened?
- Does food or liquid ever seem to come back up after swallowing? Does this ever lead to coughing or choking?
- Does the patient ever feel like meat, bread or any other foods get stuck, or cause pain in the throat or chest after swallowing?

If the patient indicates that coughing has increased in frequency, and/or that there have been incidences of choking requiring assistance, or that esophageal pain or reflux is suspected, the doctor should seriously consider a swallow study be performed. A referral can be made for follow up with a speech-language pathologist who specializes in swallow disorders or dysphagia. ASHA, the American Speech-Language-Hearing Association (asha.org), located in Rockville, Maryland, can refer you to the nearest broad-certified dysphagia specialists.

Sometimes people who have reduced sensation in the larynx do not realize they are aspirating until they develop a respiratory infection or aspiration pneumonia. Lacking laryngeal sensations or awareness to cough out intruding food or liquid is called *silent aspiration.* Anytime a pneumonia occurs in the absence of a cold or virus, aspiration should be considered. Interventions are possible for those who are experiencing diminished smelling, tasting, chewing and swallowing, but nothing can be done for a problem that isn't detected, recognized or diagnosed.

That brings us to testing. In this book's Appendix, clinicians will find a list of standardized tests for smell and taste that some ENT specialists and clinics may use. SLPs can make them a part of their cranial nerve examination. There are also informal and improvised ways to probe for deficits that can help the patients self-assess if suspecting diminished chemosensory perception. Over the rest of this chapter, the general reader will find easy- to- use formats for self-testing, each one building step by step upon the other, from *The Quick and Dirty Self-Survey* to *The Informal Self-Test.*

TESTING SMELL

SELF VS INFORMAL VS STANDARDIZED TESTS

Standardized smell tests attempt to describe and quantify the ability to detect, identify, and discriminate aromas. As such, a formal instrument has the precision to lend itself to comparisons, whether for statistical, diagnostic, or therapeutic purposes. Administering a standardized test in a sample population versus a control group can give us data on the prevalence of a disorder. In a clinician's hands, it can tell us whether a patient's performance falls within the norm or indicates a deficit. Once a deficit is identified, repeating the test can show us whether the person has improved over time due to spontaneous recovery or any intervention.

While lacking the precision of standardization, informal and self-tests can still tell an important story.

1. They can tell you whether you perceive a specific odor or taste. Yes or no.
2. As long as the degree of loss isn't too subtle, self-testing can tell you whether your sense of smell or taste is better, worse, or unchanged over time by repeating the test. It's just an estimate, of course. But it's descriptive, and you can get a ball park picture.
3. The process of self-testing on a daily basis provides the first opportunities for sensory stimulation.
4. Finally, informal and self-tests can confirm that your suspicions warrant a visit to a Primary Care Physician (PCP) or Ear, Nose and Throat (ENT) specialist. Don't hesitate to get the medical attention you need.

Numerical scales can bring a bit of precision to the process. Rating scales are used in a variety of situations, including consumer satisfaction surveys and in medical estimations of pain intensity. Pain surveys usually use a scale of 0 to 10, with 0 equal to no pain, and 10 representing the most severe pain. But anyone who has ever participated in a consumer survey over the phone or online will recognize a numerical Likert scale that usually ranges from 1 to 5. Automated surveys often ask us to describe our satisfaction with a product or service. An example is, "please tell us how likely you are to a refer a friend to XYZ Bank. Select from 1 to indicate that you are least or not likely to refer a friend, to 5, indicating that you're very likely to refer a friend." A 10 point scale allows for more nuanced responses, so a 0-10 rating has been adopted for use here.

In terms of smell and taste testing, scales can help to estimate the magnitude of strength in the detection of an odor or taste and provides a way to compare whether the current perception is approximately better or worse than on previous attempts. That means you can compare how your sensitivity is changing from day to day, week to week, or month to month. By including numerically scaled items in the first administration of an informal or self-test, you get an approximate baseline for measuring progress.

Early intervention is best. Don't delay beginning to evaluate your sensory status. Start immediately to stimulate smell and taste. Begin here with activities that are easy to do, using materials that are handy. Just remember to make notes as you go. Writing down the results of your testing can provide important documentation of your status, feelings and impressions. Instead of vague complaints, you take specific, organized observations to share with health care providers. They will be more likely to take documented experiences seriously, and it can help them to decide on the next steps.

Ready to self-test? It's simple. Try the *Quick and Dirty Self-Survey* first. You suspect something is wrong, but it's come on suddenly, not giving you time to organize a doctor's visit or any in-depth testing. Start here.

DAY 1. THE QUICK AND DIRTY SELF-SURVEY

Start by taking note of common, scented items in your environment that you use on a daily basis. The *Quick and Dirty Self-Survey* is the first day's activity. It involves working with the familiar aromas of items you have on hand. No shopping. No hassle. Everyone has objects that are scented or have aroma. Get yourself a small notebook, a notepad, staple single sheets of paper together, or create digital notes on a mobile device. Write down the name of each item you attempt to smell. Then jot down your responses to the questions posed in the text box on the opposite page. This self-survey can be completed in a single day.

Breakfast Examples

—Start with toast. Can you smell it?

—What does coffee brewing smell like? Can you smell it? Is it pleasant or unexpectantly foul-smelling?

—Open a shampoo bottle. Can you smell the liquid?

—How about scented soaps? Can you smell those?

—Open spice jars, nutmeg, cinnamon, or clove. Open a package of cheese, slice an orange. Take a whiff. Sniff any other foods you may have in your home.

Use this format to record which items you try and your responses.

Name of item	Can smell it?	Weaker?/Different?/Intensity 0-10

Write down the name of the items. Can you smell them? Yes/No

Is it weaker or unchanged in strength? On a scale of 0-10 with 0 being no perceived smell, 1-9 ranging from weakness to strength of the scent, and 10 being normal intensity, same strength as before loss, how strong (intense) is the scent? Or is intensity not an issue. Is the scent just different? Odd or atypically unpleasant or unrecognizable?

Here is an example.

Name	Can smell it?	Weaker than usual?/Different?/ Intensity 0-10
Nutmeg	Yes	yes/ – – – – – – – – – – – - /4
Cheese	No	yes/ – – – - – – – – – – – /0
Orange	Yes	yes/ – – – - – – - – – – -/3—minimal, fleeting
Coffee	Yes	no / yes, smells like sewage /10

Comments:____

Continue to pick up things in your home and put them to your nose. Could be hand lotion, hair products, pull out aromatic foods, fruits, anything that has scent. Write down the name of anything you attempt to smell. Jot down your responses to the following questions as in the example above. Can you smell it? Yes or no. If the smell is different, is the scent just weaker, or does it smell unfamiliar, unlike it previously did? This is a question that may distinguish hyposmia (weak smell) from parosmia (distorted smell). In the example given, cheese elicited a 0, no smell. This is an anosmic response. The nutmeg and orange scored 4 and 3, respectively, weaker than usual, suggesting degrees of hyposmia. Are any of the scents suddenly offensive or unpleasant? This indicates parosmia, as seen in the response to coffee. In addition to these items in this first day's survey, do you ever smell things that no one else seems to? Smell hallucinations (phantosmia)? Even though this question isn't represented in the format above, make a note of any such olfactory events in the comment field.

The Quick and Dirty Self-Survey can help you begin to make sense of a situation that can be confusing and alarming. You can calmly get a grip on what's going on and launch a methodical way to approach, understand, and describe your sensory status. Roll up your sleeves and get ready to work on recovering your senses.

If you notice any difference in the way you are perceiving the common household aromas and you wish to make an appointment with your primary care physician or ENT specialist, go ahead and do that now since you may have to wait for an appointment. Meanwhile, continue testing yourself. Your sensory deficits may spontaneously recover. But if they don't, you still have the appointment. Remember that testing is stimulation. It's a way to begin healing. After *The Quick and Dirty Self-Survey* go on to *The Using-What's- Handy* Self-Test.

Each time after you do these self-tests on any given day, you can repeat sniffing the stimuli to add intentional stimulation to the session. When you sniff an item, try to remember what it used to smell like. Recall any memories or emotions the item used to bring up with the aroma. If this process seems simple, that's because it is. It may be upsetting at first if you cannot smell things as they once were. But be patient. Little by little you may spontaneously recover. And if not, or if healing seems to be taking a long time, these tests, and the exercises that follow, will show you that you may actually be making more progress than you think. And the stimulation helps you "rewire" your brain cells. You're not just passively waiting to see a doctor. You have something constructive to do while waiting.

THE USING-WHAT'S-HANDY SELF-TEST

It can take time to assemble ingredients for the *Informal Self-Test* that follows. Until then, continue to test with what you already have on hand. But now, let's organize our sensory testing materials instead of just randomly walking through your home, picking up items to sniff as you did previously in *The Quick and Dirty Self-Survey.* Doing this new self-test will give you more diagnostic information, and the sensory stimulation is therapeutic. You will be working with a small number of items and using the same ones each time. Do this self-test every day for up to two weeks. Try it at various times of the day (noting the time under the date) to see if there's any difference in the morning or evening, just after waking up or at bedtime. Provide the context of time and activities in your notes. Be careful not to confuse your nose by exposing yourself to other aromas simultaneously. Try to create the opportunity to focus on one scent at a time without distracting or competing aromas. After a few days, as you sniff the odorants and answer the questions, see if you can discover any patterns. Are there days when you can smell a little better? Are there circumstances that seem to worsen your ability? If you have a set back, do you recover the following day and continue to make progress? Be descriptive about the process. Write notes and impressions. Create a journaling process.

Prepare individual sheets of paper, use a notebook or use digital note-taking. Enter the names of the aromas you select. Choose any 4 plus 1 from the *Additional group. Choose no more than 1 per group. See which of the following ingredients you have on hand. Don't worry if you don't have all of them. It's just a way to start testing and stimulating. Place each item in a small cup or ramekin covered with tiny, pinhole-perforated foil or wax paper. Using slips of paper and adhesive tape, label the bottom of each container with the name of the item it contains.

Stimuli groups

— coffee beans

—fresh lemon or orange peel

— clove, nutmeg, or cinnamon sticks

—fresh thyme, basil, rosemary, or mint tea

—vanilla extract

*Additional—an ounce of vinegar, whiskey or vodka, or a strong menthol cough drop

*The stimulus items in the Additional group are different in that they elicit a somatosensory or trigenimal response. We'll discuss that later.

All the ingredients should be freshly prepared on the day you test to keep the strength of the aroma at the same level over time. Stay with the same items. For example, if you start with orange peel, don't switch to lemon. Don't select more than one item per group. Be sure to take a break between sniffing each scent to clear your nose in order to avoid sensory fatigue. Since you will be repeating this self-test over a series of days to compare how your ability to smell may be changing, you will add the date to the sample format we previously used. In the example below, we compared how 4 items were perceived over three days. But you can compare over any number of days you wish. As you can see, the off-smelling coffee beans on 5/17/23 smelled stronger on 5/18/23, going from an intensity of 8 to 9. It's the number on the intensity scale that enables us to compare one day to another. That way we can see if we are smelling better or worse and to what degree. With the coffee beans, it wasn't so much an issue of a weaker or stronger smell, but that a bad aroma became worse on 5/18. Looking at the vinegar, it was minimally weaker than normal for that individual. Normal would have been a 10. But from 5/17 to 5/18 and 5/19, it didn't change, remaining a 9 in strength. If we look at the lemon peel and the clove, from 5/17 to 5/18, intensity increased from 0 (no smell perceived at all) to 2 (minimal) for the lemon peel, and from 5 to 6 for the clove. That suggested that smell had improved for those two aromas. But then on 5/19, they were perceived as weaker again, back to intensities of 0 and 5, respectively. Over a series of days, we can see whether smell is truly improving (or worsening). Perhaps, if the number only increased once, it was an atypically good day, as in the case of the lemon peel and the clove. Progress is not necessarily linear. You can leap ahead or suffer reversals in the healing process. But by comparing intensity scale numbers over time, we can see a trend. Despite set backs, you can see an overall pattern of improvement. That's the value of using a scale.

Replicate the sample format provided in the next text box. Sniff each item of your choice, then jot down your answers to the following questions.

- When you tried to smell the item, could you detect a scent? Can you smell it? Yes or No.
- Could you identify the aroma if you didn't look at it or at the label on the bottom of the cup? Yes or No.

- Does the item smell the way you remember it? Or is the smell different, even unrecognizable? Yes or No. If different, how? Try to describe it.
- Does the item smell as strong as you remember it or is it weaker? State which one. Use the 0-10 numerical scale to indicate intensity. 0—cannot smell at all, to 10—normal strength.
- Are any of the scents particularly offensive or sickening? Yes or no. If yes, which ones? Describe it in a few words. Use the comment field to further describe it or make any observations.
- At the end of the days of self-testing, note the date and summarize your results. Compare day to day, week to week. Describe any trends. Improvement? No change? Worse? Be specific.

Sample Format

Date	Name of item	Can smell it?	Identifiable?	Weaker/Different/Intensity
5/17/23	coffee beans	yes	no	——/smells like dirt——/8
Time	lemon peel	no	no	yes/——————————/0
7am	clove	yes	yes	yes/——————————/5
	vinegar	yes	yes	minimally yes/————/9

Comments: ugh! coffee beans smell weird. couldn't identify them until I looked at the label. Couldn't detect lemon peel at all.

5/18/23	coffee beans	yes	no	————/moldy dirt——/9
9:30 am	lemon peel	yes	yes	yes/——————————/2
	clove	yes	yes	yes/——————————/6
	vinegar	yes	yes	same/—————————/9

Comments: ah! i could faintly smell the lemon peel today. can't believe how bad the coffee beans smell. even worse today.

5/19/23	coffee beans	yes	no	————/moldy dirt——/9
8 am	lemon peel	yes	yes	yes/——————————/0
	clove	yes	yes	yes/——————————/5
	vinegar	yes	yes	same/—————————/9

Comments: oh, no! lost the lemon peel smell again. coffee beans still disgusting.

Date: / / Summary: Describe smell perception changes since beginning of testing.

INFORMAL SELF-TEST FOR SMELL

GATHERING MATERIALS

While beginning with what is on hand in the Using-What's-Handy Self-Test, over that week or two, you can plan and organize for the next level of self-assessment and longer-term stimulation that will follow in the training and therapy chapter. You should be able to get all you need from your local health food shop or online. You will be putting together a kit of ingredients to be placed in jars. The contents will include a variety of particular flavor aromas and essential oils.

Start with the following essential oils and aromas:

- Vanilla extract
- Rose oil (If allergic, substitute another floral, such as lilac or jasmine.)
- Eucalyptus oil or menthol cough drops
- Herbal: fresh basal, *mint, or rosemary
- Spice: whole clove, nutmeg or cinnamon stick
- Lemon oil or orange oil

*Mint oil or strong mint tea are acceptable

YOU WILL ALSO NEED:

- Dry, unscented, cotton makeup remover-type pads or cotton balls.
- Small, 1 or 2 oz, jars with lids to slow evaporation. Jars should be made of amber, green, or red glass, or hard, odorless plastic. Buy a half dozen jars to start.
- Small return address labels, or pre-cut slivers of paper, and clear adhesive tape to stick labels to the bottom of the jars
- A dark ink pen or slim-tipped marker for labeling

PREPARING THE INFORMAL SELF-TEST FOR SMELL

Place a cotton pad or ball in each jar. Sprinkle a few drops of one scent on the cotton pad or ball, then place the lid on the jar. Write the name of each aroma on a label or small slip of paper, and use the adhesive tape to stick it on the bottom of its jar. Do the same for each scent.

Several of the essential oils were originally recommended by Dr. Thomas Hummel. Hummel's classic smell training using 4 basic scents was adopted by others, including researchers, as well as *AbScent* and *Fifth Sense*. Hummel's original stimuli were expanded to 12 aromas by Altundag et al (2015, 2022) for their Modified Olfactory Training studies. I've added more options for aromatic stimuli.

Instructions:

As previously, you will be using a notebook, paper, or be making electronic notes. Copy the sample format below. There is one change from the previous format. Here, you will not write the name to the immediate right of the date. Without looking at the name of each jar, you will open it and take a short sniff, followed by a slow, long whiff. Rest your nose and sniff again. You will answer the question, can you smell it? Yes or no. For the next column you will see if you can guess the name. Got it? Then flip over the jar and see what the actual name is on the label. Enter the real name under *Name it*. Did you guess it correctly? Enter C for correct and X for incorrect. The final column is exactly as in the previous format. Decide if the scent is weaker than normal, Yes or No; if different, describe what it smells like; then estimate the strength or intensity of the scent using a scale from 0 (no smell) to 10 (normal intensity), with 1 through 9 stating how weak to strong the intensity is. If you smell nothing, state *no*, then check the label on the bottom of the jar and enter the name and either a ? or an X. Since you cannot smell it at all, you enter *Yes* under *Weaker.* Then enter a 0—no smell, under *Intensity*. Enter any descriptions or memories under *Comments*. Go through each of your aromas in the same way. Be sure to rest your nose in between. You can perform this *Informal Self-Test* once a day for as long as it takes you to recover. When you complete the day's entry, use the scents with identities now known to you to do a session of smell training. See chapter *Smell Training and Therapy: How to Do It.*

Sample Format

Date	Can smell it?Yes/No	Name it/Correct C/Incorrect X	Weaker?/Different?/Intensity(0-10)
5/21/23	Yes	lemon/ C	Yes/——————/4
	Yes	clove/ X	——/rotting weeds/9
	No	rosemary /?	Yes/——————/1
	Yes	eucalyptus/X	No/only heat felt/10
	Yes	rose/? X	Yes/—————-/ 2

Comments: The eucalyptus gave a flat irritating sensation of heat in my nose but none of the vegetal notes. The rose oil was perceived as an unidentifiable floral. Memory note: when smelling the rosemary, I couldn't recognize it but suddenly thought of my grandmother's lamb chops and Sunday dinner.

PREPARING TO PERFORM THE INFORMAL SELF-TEST

Find a quiet place, alone, without any distractions to do your sniffing for the self-test. Switch off the sound on your phone or any electronics. It's only for about 10 minutes, right? There should be no noise, music, or competing scents in the room, no room deodorizer, scented candles, cat box odors, and no food aromas. Check that you haven't put on any perfume, aftershave, scented hand lotion or scented lipstick. Make sure there is no air blowing between you and the source of the aromas.

Give yourself a quiet moment to center yourself. If you have a lot of distracting thoughts, it may help to slowly count to 10, take a breath, exhale, then proceed. Bring your nose down to the jar and take a long sniff. It may help to close your eyes as you inhale the scent in order to focus on your sense of smell and allow time for each whiff to register.

Avoid nose fatigue! Be sure to rest after taking in a few sniffs, and particularly before moving on to another scent. Some people in the perfume industry find it helpful to use a cleansing aroma, such as coffee beans, to refresh their nose. But if you have parosmia and coffee is unpleasant to smell, simply rest a couple minutes before moving on to the next scent.

TESTING TASTE

INFORMAL TASTE TESTS

Ingredients for testing the 5-basic tastes may be perishable and should be prepared fresh for immediate use. It is helpful to work with a partner and use a blind fold, but it's not absolutely necessary. Pre-mix the solutions (the taste-test stimuli) in 5 cups that have been labeled on the bottom with the words: sweet, sour, salty, bitter, umami (or savory), respectively. Each solution can be used straight from the mixing cup, or poured into and shaken in a dark colored bottle with a screw-on, eye dropper lid. Small bottles with eye dropper lids can be purchased online, at some local pharmacies, or health food stores. Make sure the bottles are glass, or food grade and scent-free hard plastic for safety. The bottles should be dark amber, green or red colored. By using tinted bottles, the taster won't see the color of coffee or broth, for example, and the name of the basic taste stimulus (bitter or umami, in this case) won't be given away.

The pre-mixed taste stimuli can be delivered to the tongue on a teaspoon or by eye dropper. Regardless of whether you work with a partner for the actual test, you will need someone who is able to taste normally to try each pre-mixed solution to be sure that the taste sample is strong enough.

Once the person indicates the strength is adequate for the sweet, salty, and umami solutions, which have been dissolved in water, keep the proportion of water to stimuli exactly the same for any subsequent retests in the future. For example, if using 1-teaspoon of sugar to 2 ounces of water, always use those exact amounts.

Ingredients. The pre-mixed taste stimuli are:

- Sweet: sucrose dissolved as sugar water
- Salty: salt (sodium chloride) dissolved in water
- Sour: citric acid (straight) or lemon juice (undiluted)
- Bitter: black coffee (straight) or (quinine) tonic water (undiluted)
- Umami/savory: unsalted beef broth, or unsalted beef bouillon, or monosodium glutamate, dissolved in a minimal amount of water.

In a notebook or journal, create and label columns in a format similar to the way you did it for the *Informal Self-Test for Smell.*

Date:__/___/___

Name	Identified? Yes/No	Weak/Distorted/ Intensity (0-10)
sweet		
sour		
salty		
bitter		
savory		
tap water (optional, as control)		

Comments:____

The taster or the partner will serve one of the 5-basic tastes. The taster will guess which of the 5-basic tastes they are experiencing: sweet, salty, sour, bitter, or umami (savory), as it's presented. Plain tap water can be used as a foil or control.

After each taste, the taster cleanses their palate with a sip of water. The taster may be able to tell what the specific substance is; for example, sour/lemon or bitter/coffee, all to the good, but that is not the immediate object of this test. The object is whether the taster can identify that the stimulus is one of the 5-basic tastes by stating the name: sweet, sour, salty, bitter, or umami (savory). To summarize: the taster should guess which of the tastes is being presented and state it. The response is written down. Then the label on the cup or bottle is checked. If the taster correctly identified the taste, then a Yes is entered, if No, then that is entered. Remember: the taster should clear their palate with a sip or two of water and wait approximately 60 seconds between each taste stimulus.

In order to track progress, this test can be repeated once a week, if any of the 5-basic tastes were undetected or incorrectly named. Be sure to use every one of the stimuli every time, and do not look at the name of the substance before tasting it. If administering the stimuli to yourself, in order to test blind, it is helpful to use the recommended amber, red, or green colored bottles with eye droppers.

TESTING FOR SOMATOSENSORY COMPONENTS OF SMELL AND TASTE

Sensory receptors in the nose, mouth and throat are designed to detect light touch, pressure, temperature and pain. These are often referred to as the trigeminal (related to the Trigeminal or Cranial Nerve V pathways) or the somatosensory aspects of taste. Some of the somatosensory receptors are situated close to the tastebuds and smell receptors, and the neural pathways sometimes run adjacent before diverging from those of smell and the 5- basic tastes. When illness or injury strikes, depending on the exact areas affected, the somatosensory pathways may be simultaneously impaired or left intact. We need to know if they are affected or not, and if so, to what degree.

Later in this book, these somatosensory sensations are referred to as the basis of "flavor element variables," because they usually accompany smell and the basic-5 tastes. In some cases, we can bypass smell and taste when those perceptions are deficient, and compensate by using somatosensory perceptions therapeutically, as well as to contribute to overall flavor impressions during actual meals.

As you work through the probes that follow, use your journal or notebook. Describe where and how you experience these sensations. For example, note whether you feel them on just the tongue? Which part? Or on the inside of your cheeks? The roof of your mouth, or the back of your throat? The more specific the description of your oral and nasal sensitivities the better. Remember that these self-tests have a diagnostic value that will enable you, or an SLP, to narrow the search when selecting the appropriate training and compensatory procedures in this book.

INFORMAL TEST FOR THE SOMATOSENSORY RECEPTORS AND PATHWAYS

In your journal or notebook, jot down the names of the substances (food stimuli) you use, and describe your reactions to each one. You want to record any substance that you were not able to feel at all (yes/no), or ones that felt diminished when compared to how you used to sense them. On a scale of 0-no sensation at all, to 10-normal sensation, record the strength of these somatosensory perceptions. Follow the instructions for Nose and Mouth/Throat, and describe your reactions by filling in the information in the *Somatosensory Self-Test* form. If any somatosensory perceptions are weak or absent, repeat the test weekly to track progress. Remember to rest your nose, and rinse your mouth and throat, after trying each stimulus.

NOSE:

Open a bottle of whiskey, vodka or gin that are 80 proof or stronger. DO NOT DRINK the alcohol.

Pass the bottle just under the nose or immerse a cotton swab in the alcohol and pass it under the nose.

Bring your nose close to the liquid just momentarily. Do you recoil from a whiff of the strong alcohol?

If not, dip a cotton swab in 70% rubbing alcohol and pass the swab under your nostrils. Did you want to pull your head back from the smell? Can you feel that the alcohol is an irritant?

Can you sense any other irritants, such as menthol in a strong menthol/eucalyptus cough drop? Do you sense it as irritant in the nose or when in the mouth? Wasabi can be substituted for a cough drop.

MOUTH AND THROAT:

Temperature: Take a sip of hot coffee, tea or any other hot liquid. Test it to be sure it isn't hot enough to burn you.

Can you sense the heat of a hot beverage on your tongue?

Place an ice chip on your tongue. Can you feel the cold of the ice?

Texture: Can you feel the smoothness of yogurt? The crunchiness of toast? The chewy sensations of a piece of fruit roll, taffy, or a piece of steak or chicken?

Astringency: Are you able to feel the drying or puckering sensation from a drop of lemon or vinegar?

Spicy burn: Place 1/4 teaspoon of tabasco sauce or chili sauce on your tongue. Move the substance around in your mouth. Can you feel any burn? Where? Rinse with cool water or yogurt.

Light touch: Brush your tongue with a sprig of parsley, or drag dental floss across your tongue. Right side, left, front, back. Any place on your tongue that you couldn't feel it?

Pressure: Can you feel the weight of an ice cube, a melon ball, or a teaspoon of peanut butter on your tongue?

Note on Pressure: Clinicians have a variety of instruments and ways to assess sensitivity to light and deep touch. Essentially, we want to know if you can feel a gentle stroke or the weight of a particular food/liquid. Sensing of pressure is important for manipulating substances in the mouth so that a bolus of food is prepared and can trigger a swallow. Pressure perception is related to texture. Texture is also related to proprioception, the ability to sense movement, force, and position of muscles and joints, but this topic isn't essential to our discussion here.

Somatosensory Self-Test

Date: __/__/__

Nose	Yes/No	Intensity of Sensation (1-10)
alcohol		
menthol		
wasabi		

Comments:____

Mouth/Throat	Substance	Yes/No	Intensity of Sensation(1-10)
temperature			
texture			
astringency			
burn (spicy)			
light touch			
pressure			

Comments:___________________________________

WHAT IS THE NATURE OF YOUR SENSORY DEFICIT?

After using the informal self-tests even once, you will have a better idea whether your problem is smell, taste, or a combination of both. You'll also know whether your somatosensory receptors and pathways are intact. This information is essential for guiding the reader through these pages in order for you to create a relevant self-training. It's also key for clinicians designing specific, patient-centered rehabilitation.

Listed in the Appendix are the names of formal tests that might be encountered in a medical or research setting.

Speech-language pathologists can also acquire the formal tests. Given what the pandemic has taught us about viruses and the loss of smell and taste, I strongly recommend that SLPs integrate smell and taste tests, whether formal or informal, as supplementary probes along with traditional cranial nerve or oral-peripheral speech mechanism and swallowing examinations. SLPs should test the smell, taste and trigeminal pathways. They may be familiar with testing the trigeminal pathways as it relates to touch, but hopefully the SLPs reading this book can see that it's more complicated than that when it comes to motivating dysphagic patients with dysosmia and dysgeusia. Consider additional probes suggested in the informal somatosensory testing just described. You may not be able to do it all in one session, but I assure you, it can make a huge difference in designing therapy. An important note for clinicians: Do not use alcoholic beverages to test for smell irritant. Even though, of course, you will not ask the patient to drink it, your intentions might be misconstrued. Instead, use rubbing alcohol on a cotton swab and pass it under the nose.

SUMMARIZING YOUR TESTING RESULTS

Now that you've tested your sense perceptions, it's recommended that you summarize your findings and have them at the ready. You'll need to create a verbal composite of your strengths and deficits. You can transfer your findings from all the self-tests and consolidate them onto one easy-to- view master summary sheet (page 91).

For the column on the left labeled Smell, Taste, and Somatosensory, use a checkmark to indicate that you were able to smell, taste or feel the particular item. Use the initials N, A, W, D to indicate whether the perception was normal, absent, weak or distorted, respectively. Use the Intensity scale numbers from the tests to fill out the + 0-10 column. Be sure you make room to describe the nature of the perception.

Number 5 asks you to try to analyze which foods or beverages are particularly problematic and see if you can identify the component flavors or aromas that may be the offenders. For example, beef stew. Analyze the component parts: browned meat, onion, gravy, potato, carrot. Rinse off each one, then sniff or taste again. Which component seems to be the problem? It may take several trials to find a pattern of flavors or aromas that need to be reduced or eliminated from your diet or disguised. Eliminated foods might be slowly reintroduced over time through desensitization. Also, this exercise will help you identify foods and aromas that are actually acceptable when isolated from that particular dish. Finding those acceptable foods can make a world of difference.

Testing Summary

1. Smell Normal/Absent/Weak/Distorted/+ 0-10

Citrus

Floral

Resinous

Spice

Herbal

Other aromas (Specify)

2. Taste Normal/Absent/Weak/Distorted/+ 0-10

Sweet

Salty

Sour

Bitter

Umami

3. Somatosensory Normal/Absent/Weak/Distorted/+0-10

Textures:

smooth

oily

wet

slippery

crunchy

chewy

creamy

buttery

other

Light touch/stroke

Pressure

Temperature Hot___ Cold___

Pain/Burn

Meal Time Observations

4. Foods/Beverages that are unpleasant or intolerable;

____

____

5.Component flavors that are suspected offenders in #4:

____

____

SEVEN

SMELL TRAINING AND THERAPY: HOW TO DO IT.

Smell training has been recommended for many, varying causes of sensory loss. To me, the term *training* is problematic. Smell or taste training was something I, as a professional taster, with my chemosensory facilities intact, did for many years. I did not have to rehabilitate lost senses. But that is exactly what many reading this book *must* do. When we train, we go from a normal but unskilled state to a skilled one. When we lose an ability, we rehabilitate to restore or approximate a normal or pre-morbid condition. Rehabilitation requires therapy. That assumes the provider of the therapy is educated in the mechanisms underlying normal and disordered (sensory) function, as well as being knowledgable, certified, and skilled in techniques to rehabilitate the individual with the disorder. This book is a general guide that instructs patients and caregivers how to apply rehabilitative techniques after they define their sensory deficits using the self-assessments, and work through the exercises and suggestions offered. However, a patient may need an approach better targeted to their individual symptoms and challenges. They may need someone to fine tune or problem solve with them. And this is where an objective professional, such as an SLP, if trained in the science of smell and taste, can be of great assistance.

It's possible to hit road blocks, to feel overwhelmed, and to become discouraged by a general guide. A professional therapist can help break down the rehabilitative steps into small, attainable goals, thus preventing stagnation and frustration. A clinician can provide perspective and encouragement when the patient may feel discouraged. The professional can use this book as a starting point, then follow the evolving research that can shed light on options, insights, expectations and the latest techniques. Just as this book is no substitute for medical intervention, it is also not a substitute for a licensed therapist who has educated themselves in the olfactory and degustatory science.

If professional assistance is needed, it can take time to find someone qualified. Meanwhile, patients and caregivers cannot afford to do nothing. Engage with this book to the best of your ability. Once a smell or tasting loss is discovered, we should waste no time in stimulating those senses. The sooner the better, even if the usual period for spontaneous recovery has not expired. The reason is simple. The fresher the memory of smell or taste or flavor, the more available it will be to remind our brain cells. Evoking a memory that is fresh, vivid, and detailed is easier to reinforce and to bring to new smelling and tasting opportunities. We want to take advantage of these recent memories, as well as long term ones, to help establish new neural connections and minimize any damage.

TRAINING IS A SLOW RECOVERY MARATHON, NOT A SPRINT!

Think of how a healthy person exercises to get into shape. It's an organized effort in which they master the same exercises, perform the same number of repetitions, then increase the variety of exercises over time. They step up to more reps, heavier weights or increased resistance in a systematic way. If you never worked out at the gym or with weights, maybe you've run or walked for fitness. It's still organized and methodical. There's usually a procedure. Run or walk a minimum number of times a week. Maybe start at 20 minutes. Stretch. Cool down afterwards. Soon you're doing 30 minutes. Work up to walking or running a mile, then a mile and a half, then two miles. Maybe go a full hour. The point is, to get results, we need to approach training in a systematic manner. You will do the same with smell and taste training or therapy.

Only one caveat. When working on an exercise program, we are healthy people. It is a goal to push our limits. By doing so intelligently, injury and exhaustion can be avoided. But a person recovering from a virus or a traumatic injury is not starting with health. That person must take care not to stress, not to push, not to re-injure. Work must be slower, subtler, more deliberate. It may seem too slow at times, as if you're hardly doing anything, barely moving forward. Patience! What may take a few months for some can take a year, even two or more for others.

Respect your own process. Compare yourself with no one. There's no way to control the time it will take. Let go of any timetable in your mind. Goals involving time are artificial constructs. They are goal posts that often have to be moved.

Your healing is unique and will take whatever time it takes. Just start! Take one small step in the healing direction. Your objective is not about speed, but what it might be to smell anything, to smell more, to smell or taste better, to slow down the loss of a sense in the case of a degenerating illness, or to be able to compensate when total recovery may not be possible.

Your job is to stimulate and make notes. You will retest from time to time to create some measure of your progress. And you'll continue on, stimulating. Communicate your needs. Practice patience, self-love, self-forgiveness, and optimism, even if those are foreign concepts for you. And if you accomplish any of those mental attitudes, you will be growing, learning, and healing, at least on a psychological level. And that's good in itself. Because there's no physical healing without movement in mental well-being.

Okay, you've done the self-assessment in the previous chapter. Now let's prepare stimulation kits.

START WITH WHAT YOU HAVE

Construct an aroma stimulation kit from your pantry. Maybe you're still not feeling well enough to go out to shop. It takes time to assemble a smell training/therapy kit, whether putting it together as a do-it-yourself project described in this book, or by ordering ones pre-made. As previously stated, it's best not to lose time waiting for the perfect smell training kit. You may already have some of the ingredients left over from your self-testing that can be repurposed here for the smell training/therapy. In addition, use the previously introduced self-testing format (below) in a journal or as electronic notes to track your training/therapy progress.

Date	Name of item	Can smell it?	Identifiable?	Weaker?/Different?/Intensity0-10
—/—/—				
Time				
:				
am/pm				

Comments: ______________________________

Let's start by opening your kitchen pantry and refrigerator. You will need a knife, cutting board, small ziplock snack bags, small cups or ramekins, and foil, wax paper, or plastic wrap. Later, as soon you order and receive them, you can transfer smell stimuli to the 1-2 oz colored glass or scent-free hard plastic jars, as described in the testing chapter. After the first week or two, you should also shift from highly perishable items to essential oils which are long lasting.

Assemble as many of the smell stimuli items as possible. Choose one from each group below and stick with it. In other words, don't switch from one type citrus to another, or one type herb or spice to another, at least not right away. You can add others later, but don't use them interchangeably. The main thing is to be consistent and organized.

PREPARE SMELL STIMULI

1. Citrus fruit: orange, lemon, lime, or grapefruit. Choose only one!

Citrus fruits have wonderful aromas, both in the body of the fruit and the peel. These are common scents that most people with intact smelling readily recognize. When we peel an orange, the rind contains oils that retain the scent and remain on our fingers, requiring an effort to remove. The aromas of lemon and orange are commonly available as essential oils and are also sold as flavorings in the cooking ingredients aisles of grocery stores. Try to get the essential oil or flavor additive versions as soon as possible. Check the expiration dates and ask people with normal smell perception to confirm that the aromas retain a fully potent and typical smell.

But you can start now, if you already have citrus in your home. Choose one type of citrus fruit and slice it into small sections. Peel off the rind of one section and store the rest of the sections away for future use. Place the rind of the one section in a small snack bag and zip it shut, or roll it into tin foil or plastic wrap. Every day, or at least every other day, change to a fresh peel from another section. You should have enough to last a week.

2. Cinnamon, nutmeg or clove.

Sticks and whole forms are preferable. Ground forms can lose strength, and you have to be careful not to inhale the powder. Place a stick of cinnamon, or whole nutmeg or clove, in a snack bag, or use the jar in which it comes. You do not need to switch to an essential oil or flavoring for these spices if you use them in their whole forms. They last a long time. The spice should be recently purchased to be optimally potent. If ground, ask someone if the scent seems to be full strength.

3. Fresh herbs such as mint, rosemary, oregano, thyme or basil. Keep them rolled in a paper towel in the refrigerator. They are highly perishable, of course. Thyme, oregano, basil and rosemary can sometimes be found in small plastic boxes in the market. I've purchased these and found that they have remained aromatic in their original packaging for a couple weeks. In their dried forms, they may not much resemble the fresh. Place a few fresh sprigs of one herb type in the snack bag each day and seal it. If you have mint tea bags instead of fresh mint, you can use that if recently purchased and it retains full potency. Check the expiration date, and ask someone with intact smelling to check that the tea bags have a good, strong aroma.
4. Anything floral. It could be in an essential oil, a floral perfume, or a floral scented soap, shampoo or hand cream. Perfumes can be complex because they are composites of many aromatic notes. Perfume manufacturers often license shampoo makers to use their scents in hair products. So the same warnings may apply as to perfumes. Citrus and spice notes are common in perfumes and we want to avoid those since we are already using isolated citrus and spices. Choose a perfume that has dominant notes of rose, ylang ylang, or gardenia, if you have one. Start with what's on hand, but it's best to obtain the pure essential oils. Short term, a scented soap may work. A favorite soap from my childhood was classic Camay®

which smells like honeysuckle. Many other soaps contain dominant lavender or other floral notes. Soap can be cut into pieces or placed whole in snack bags right out of their wrappers. Vanilla is both a flower and a spice. The extract contains some alcohol but once dropped onto the cotton pad, it will likely evaporate.

5. Eucalyptus essential oil, or menthol cough drops, if strongly scented. These aromas, in addition to the olfactory nerve, trigger the trigeminal pathway which conveys heat and irritants in certain kinds of volatiles, such as alcohol. It's helpful to know that the receptors and pathways are intact. We already had you test yourself by sniffing whiskey or rubbing alcohol to see if your nose reacts to them as irritants. But our purpose is different here. Eucalyptus and menthol have more than just heat. If you sense vegetal aromas in the eucalyptus, and more in the cough drops beyond the heat, it is important to note that, as this can suggest ways to compensate for missing flavor during recovery.
6. Coffee beans. As an optional, additional aroma. Some people with parosmia find coffee foul-smelling. It may be tempting to exclude it from daily exposure. But unless it causes severe reactions, work with it, particularly if you were an enthusiastic coffee drinker. Place a dozen beans in a snack bag and use it to desensitize yourself to any unpleasantness with tiny, fleeting exposures. Use it for memory work as described later.

Now that you have assembled your short-term, homemade smell training/therapy kit, how do you use it?

SMELL TRAINING/ THERAPY PROCEDURE

Use this procedure for all training/therapy, whether the kits assembled were self-made or ordered pre-made. Select convenient times of the day so you can make sensory stimulation part of your daily routine. You might do it for a few minutes when you first wake up, or just before you're about to brush your teeth in the evening. Select times around activities you do every day so it's easy to remember to also do the smell therapy. Start with just a 10-minute session, at least twice a day. That includes smelling and writing any notes. If you can spare more time, great! If you can do a smell session three times a day, excellent! But avoid too many repetitions without resting the nose. Remember, the nose can fatigue and needs time to reset.

PREPARE THE ENVIRONMENT.

- Use a fan, open window, or air conditioner to ventilate the room to remove any ambient smells, such as coffee or cooking odors or room fresheners. Remove scented hand cream or lipstick, or any odors that could compete with the target aromas.
- Set up a tray of the scent stimuli, set them next to a chair or on the nightstand next to your bed. Keep the stimuli out of direct sunlight.
- Notebook, journal or electronic device (audio off!) ready?

- Turn off your phone and any noise, music, radio or television. You will need to be alone and distraction-free for those 10-20 minutes.

BEGIN SMELL TRAINING/THERAPY

1. Sit down. Clear your mind of any distracting thoughts. If it helps to center yourself, take a breath, exhale fully once, focus by counting slowly to 10 in order to clear your mind, take another breath and exhale, then…
2. Open the first container of scent stimuli. Lower your nose to the opened container. Take a short sniff. Exhale. Could you smell anything? Could you identify what it was without looking at it?
3. Take another sniff of the same scent, this time a longer whiff, and allow any sensory or emotional memories connected to the aroma to surface.
4. Count to 10 to clear your mind. Say the name of the aroma and take one more long sniff to connect to any memories and sensory impressions. Close the container.
5. Rest your nose for about 60 seconds. Use the time to make your journal, notebook or digital notes. Record your impressions. Use the format provided earlier in this chapter. Answer the following questions.

- Were you able to smell anything? Yes/No
- Were you able to identify the scent without looking at the name?Yes/No

- Did the scent seem true to its identity or distorted? Describe any distortion.
- Did the scent seem full strength or weaker than usual?
- On a scale of 0 (no aroma) to 10 (normal strength) rate the intensity of the aroma.

Entry complete, go on to the next aroma. Repeat these 5 steps, including the journal entry, for each of the scent stimuli.

After the first week, review the journal entries, particularly the intensity scale column, to compare day to day performance. Review comments to note any change. Make note of any trends, progress, reversals. Use the comment field to describe any changes.

If you do not fully recover your sense of smell and taste within 2-4 weeks, it is recommended that you move on to longer-term Smell Training/Therapy. Most people recover within a short time, but let's prepare for the "just in case" scenario. A small percentage of people may not see improvement until after 8 months. Progress can be unpredictable and vary with each individual, so make the procedure part of your life, and be patient for results. You may see progress, then have days of no advance or even regression. Stress and fatigue or other illnesses can cause such fluctuations. Don't be discouraged. Progress often continues after a set back. Above all, be patient. Don't abandon the practice!

Make note of changes, even subtle ones. Writing in the journal is important. It can seem like you're getting nowhere because you may compare how you are to the way things used to be before you lost your smell or taste. But when you read your journal entries, you might be surprised that there has indeed been some progress. Gains can be subtle. You might not even notice them without reading back your journal notes or retesting. So don't skip the journal writing or the retesting.

Keep up the good work!

ASSEMBLING A CLASSIC OR MODIFIED SMELL TRAINING/THERAPY KIT

You can purchase ready-made smell training kits, such as those available through abscent.org. But if you don't live in the UK, it may be quicker and less costly to simply make your own. And it's easy. Here's how.

- If you haven't ordered them yet, buy a half dozen, 1or 2 ounce colored jars with lids. Amber, red or green glass or hard, unscented plastic jars are inexpensive and easy to order online. The reason for the color is so that light does not alter the contents, also so that you are not cued to the name of the scent by any visual information.
- Buy blank, small return address-size labels. Or make your own using slips of paper and clear adhesive tap. Write down the name of each scent stimulus on a label or slip of paper and stick them on the bottom of a jar. One name to each jar.
- Buy unscented, cotton makeup remover pads or cotton balls. Saturate a couple pads or a cotton ball with one essential oil, place in a jar, screw on the lid, stick a label the bottom of the jar with the name of the scent. Repeat for each of the scents.

- Buy essential oils from health food stores or online. Hummel's basic 4 were rose, lemon, eucalyptus and clove. He described these as floral, fruity, resinous, and spicy.

What if you have allergies to one of the Hummel 4? You can substitute other essential oil scents; such as, lilac, jasmine, geranium or ylang ylang instead of rose; orange or grapefruit oil instead of lemon; pine instead of eucalyptus; all spice or nutmeg instead of clove. Whichever ones you select, stick to the same 4 for the first 3 months.

Use the Smell Training/Therapy Procedure introduced earlier in this chapter for each session and the Begin Smell Training/ Therapy steps for each of the scents. Begin with the 4 scents. Refresh them with a couple new drops every week. Practice at least 2 times a day.

The stimuli were originally meant to be used for 4-6 months. Altundag et al. (2022), for their study of post-COVID sufferers of parosmia, modified the smell training procedures to add 4 new stimuli every 12 weeks for a total of 36 weeks. Significant gains were noted during the final 3 months for those with long COVID parosmia. However, people can continue to improve long after.

Here is the order Altundag's team used:

Weeks 1 - 12: (Hummel) eucalyptus, lemon, rose, and clove.

Next 12 weeks: menthol, tangerine, thyme and jasmine.

Last 12 weeks: green tea, bergamot, rosemary, and gardenia

You can continue to use the Hummel 4 after the first 12 weeks, or add new items, as Altundag's group did, at 12 weeks, 24 weeks and 36 weeks. Changing keeps the process interesting. You can do a weekly self-test to see how you have progressed. If your perception of these aromas isn't totally restored by 9 months, please don't get discouraged. Keep stimulating. Contrary to previous thinking that people reached their limits for improvement at 1 year, gains even after 2 years are possible.

EVOKING MEMORY IN SMELL AND TASTE THERAPY

If you want to sell a house, it has been suggested by some realtors to fill your home with the scent of baking cookies or hot apple cider with cinnamon. The savvy agents are trying to evoke in the prospective buyer powerful, childhood sensory memories. There are good physiological and psychological reasons underlying this sales strategy. Emotional and sensory memories are often coded together, and the location of these memories interact with centers of decision making. The delicious aromas of the cookies or cider give rise to feelings that correspond to all that the concept of home embodies: nourishment, love, belonging, security, safety. These are strong emotions. And these feelings drive motivation to action, in the case of real estate, the purchasing of a home.

Advertising people know that emotions and motivation drive actions. Politicians know that. Unless we're aware that they are pulling our emotional strings, we will act as unthinking marionettes. Even the most prudent among us have all made impulsive purchases. We've all been manipulated. Open your closet or refrigerator. Bet you'll find plenty of evidence.

Advertising often operates by making us feel inadequate in some way, then proposes a solution in the form of a product. Aromas orchestrated by savvy marketers are aimed at evoking emotions and thoughts that will make us feel more attractive, lovable, or socially acceptable. The product marketing seems to say, "here's what you're missing: family, warmth, happy gatherings. We can give you the things you lack, or some facsimile thereof." Walk into the cosmetic department of a store, a housewares department. They're loaded with scent. One sniff and they're betting you'll take the product home. Walk into a hotel. Many have proprietary scents designed for them by fragrance companies. Each sniff evokes a signature mood. Their goal is to turn you into a repeat customer. If there is any silver lining to the cloud of anosmia, perhaps it's being less vulnerable to manipulation through the nose. But, of course, the predominant emotion for most anosmics and parosmics is not relief. Most would be willing to risk a bit of manipulation for restored smell perception.

Many reading this book know well how the loss of smell can deprive us of accessing emotional memories. A dimension of our everyday lives is lost. The world is flat, or flatter, at least. We go for a walk and feel the breeze on our faces. But where is the scent of apple blossoms in the spring, lilac trees and rose gardens, the mulch of autumn, that crisp nostril-kiss of an imminent winter snow? Right in this moment, as you read these words, your mind is trying to recall such scents. The words trigger a desire to imagine. Hold onto that fact! The willingness to imagine is a decision made in a nanosecond. You just did it! Without even realizing it.

We can make this process conscious and deliberate. A choice. You can decide to call up sense memories to work for you in smell and taste therapy too. Just as a loss of sensory input can deprive us of memories, we can marshal memories to reconnect us to the world of smell and taste. Just turn on your imagination! You already did it reading this, so you know how to do it. The will to imagine hasn't been lost to disease. Just as you can read words to evoke smell memories, you can use the associated emotions to help rebuild the neural networks of sensory perception.

Here's how to do it!

MEMORY EVOKING EXERCISES FOR SMELL

1. Let's use our other senses to help us recall a vivid smell memory. It could be something from childhood, for example, a delicious cooking aroma or scents from nature and the outdoors. If not from childhood, a smell memory could be something in the recent past, before you lost your ability to smell. Close your eyes, and without trying to evoke the smell itself, picture in your mind the circumstances of the smell memory you wish to recall. Where were you? Recall details of the place. Visualize the surroundings. Recall who was with you, if anyone at all. Make the visual aspects vivid and detailed. What were you wearing? What kind of day was it? What objects were in the environment? Zoom in on details. What colors can you recall? What sounds did you hear? Recall the instant you detected the smell. And most important, what emotions were you feeling? What did the smell make

you feel? Let the memory of the aroma come flooding back. As if turning up the volume on a radio, turn up the smell in your memory. Make the smell memory so loud that you cannot hear or see anything else. Zoom in on that smell memory so that it's so large, you cannot see anything else. Hold that a moment, then let it go. Great work!

2. Now let's apply the same memory technique to an aroma of a specific food or scent item that is absent, diminished or distorted today. Close your eyes. Think of an item you used to perceive as particularly pleasant. It could be coffee, chocolate, or a juicy steak, as a food. Or it could be a favorite perfume or a flower. Whatever it might be that is disconcerting now because it is offensive or undetectable to you. Don't focus on the smell memory yet. Let's try to call up every other sensory detail surrounding that particular moment. Recall the last time the smell was pleasant, even adored. You can start with an emotion or visual detail of that last wonderful smell encounter. Try to connect with the emotion. Name that emotion. Try to recall what you saw. Zoom in on every visual and auditory detail, every leaf on a tree or pattern on wallpaper, colors, voices, sounds, even items you may have touched. Connect with the emotion you felt while enjoying the aroma at that particular time. Try to zoom in on the emotion as if it you could increase the loudness on a volume control, enlarge the emotion as if using the lens of a camera. Now, using your imagination and memory try to smell the aroma of the item as it was then. Can you

recall it? If so, turn up the volume, zoom in on that scent memory. Excellent!

Repeat this exercise every day for several days. Then take the next step.

3. Superimposing scent memories over the current absent or distorted smells.

   Begin by selecting an actual item to work on. A favorite food or scent. Don't touch it yet. Don't attempt to smell it. Perform #2 of the Memory Evoking Exercises with the favorite food or scent in mind. When your memory of the details, and especially the emotions, surrounding that pleasant smelling event are most vivid, with the emotional and smell memories loudest in volume,or maximally zoomed in, take a whiff of the actual item you wish to smell as you used to do. As you inhale, superimpose the sensory memory over the current smell. Keep turning up the volume of the formerly pleasant memory so that any aroma absence or distortion in the present moment is drowned out by the memory. Hold that zoomed memory as you inhale for about 5 seconds. Then remove the item from your field of smell and rest your nose.

Don't be surprised if you feel mentally tired from these exercises. On the other hand, you may feel rejuvenated. Regardless, take a break. Rest your senses and your mind. You can repeat the exercises later. At a minimum, try to do #2 and #3 of the *Memory Evoking Exercise* twice a day after the smell therapy exercises described previously in this chapter.

PROCEDURE:

- Complete the smell training/therapy session including journal entry for the 4 aromas as you now do every day.
- Select one of the aromas to use for emotional memory work.
- When you complete turning up the volume as in #3, take a whiff of the actual aroma,
- and now use the intensity scale again to rate the strength of the aroma.

Fill in the journal form, adding the new Memory Evoking section.

Date Name of item Can smell it? Identifiable? Weaker?/Different?/Intensity (0-10)

—/—/—

Time

:

am/pm

Comments: ____

Memory Evoking: I worked with (Name of aroma) ________________

When I did memory work with ______ the aroma was perceived at ______ level of intensity.

Was there any change between the first attempt to smell the aroma and the attempt during the memory evoking work? Yes/No

Comment: ____

EIGHT

REHABILITATION OF TASTE AND FLAVOR

What we generally consider *taste* is actually *flavor*, a composite of smell (retronasal), the 5-basic tastes, and somatosensory perceptions. When we bite into a piece of chocolate then ride out the smoothness as it melts, cool down to the chill of ice cream, warm to a steamy hot chocolate, or wince from the burn of an excessively spicy chili, we can thank our somatosensory pathways. When we push the concept of texture to include the consuming of chewy taffy or crunchy tortilla chips without biting our tongue, the proprioceptive pathways kick in.

As essential as this proprioception is to the mechanics of chewing and swallowing, most of us would not consider the sensing and regulation of muscle and joint movements as integral to flavor as the somatosensory perceptions of temperature, touch, pressure or pain.

We can to a large degree separate those proprioceptive processes from the actual perception of flavor. Vision and hearing are different, however, and seem to contribute more to the sense of flavor, despite being more peripheral. Think about how, without seeing the color red, you might not find the flavor of a pale pink strawberry so vibrant. The paleness suggests you anticipate the berry as less sweet, and the flavor-creating brain will oblige. Now consider a potato chip without a crunchy sound. You'd find it stale. Food producers spend fortunes on science and marketing. They know that input which has nothing to do with the nose or mouth still influences our impressions of flavor and our desire to consume their particular brands.

Smell training involves the orthonasal route, where volatile molecular compounds of odorants are inhaled, whether passively or actively, and are taken up by receptor cells in the mucosal, or epithelial, lining of the nasal passages. Chemical signals are generated via the nerve endings then fed directly to the brain's first way station, the olfactory bulb. Then the signal goes to various points along the olfactory pathway, triggering detection thresholds and recognition mechanisms while interacting with emotional memory and qualitative judgements. It's amazingly complex, yet takes place within nanoseconds.

But the perception of flavor adds retronasal smell to the mix, as the molecules of odorants are released during chewing and exhaling, transformed in the mucosal receptors along the way, then too are routed to the olfactory bulb of the brain.

We also know that the pathways of the basic-5 tastes and the sensations of pressure, touch, temperature, and pain travel to the brain stem, then are relayed to the cerebral cortex where they eventually link up to the olfactory signals. The olfactory and taste pathways route through centers that specialize in memory, emotion, and hedonic (pleasure/displeasure) value assignment, and meet up with the signals sent along the somatosensory pathways. These complex reactions happen far more quickly than the conscious mind can ever register. And it is through the integration of all these impulses in the brain that flavor is created. This brain-created flavor perception is why I emphasize the importance of therapy that includes the integration of smell, taste, and somatosensory perceptions along with other sensory and emotional memories to fully recover our ability to experience flavor.

A LOOK AT INTEGRATED THERAPY

- Smell is an integral step in preparing us to receive food. Smell triggers the production of saliva, essential to breaking down food into digestible molecules and nutrients. When smell is not accessible, we need other ways to prepare the mouth and digestive system.
- Memory and imagination, along with the direct stimulation (e.g., tongue stroking) of the somatosensory pathways, can help produce saliva.
- When smell is not accessible, we can call upon the 5-basic tastes and oral sensations via somatosensory impulses to fill out an impression of flavor. We use what we can. That means we need our teeth to bite, our jaw muscles to flex and release in order to chew, our tongues to transport food and liquid to back of the mouth and to trigger swallowing. We need to

perceive muscle flexion, movement and pressure for swallowing and a sense of texture, temperature, and pain (burn) to approximate flavor. We need to bring in memory and emotion. And to maximize the experience, it helps to toss visual and auditory stimuli into the mix.

BREATHING AND FLAVOR

When we chew and our saliva mixes with food, we prepare the digestive tract for swallowing as we form, then move, a food bolus towards the back of the mouth, the oropharynx. We don't stop breathing during all this but are intermittently inhaling and exhaling, and as we do, aromas rise up through the space between the soft palate and the back of the nasal passages (the retronasal pathway). Ever have something you're drinking rush out your nose? The architectural structure of the retronasal pathway is the exit route.

Complex coordination prepares us to hold our breath in order to protect our airway from aspiration as we swallow. Except for that rare event of beer or soda snorting while we laugh, this maneuver usually works. With the soft palate shielding the nasopharyngeal space, the food bolus or liquid is propelled from the back of the tongue over a chute-like structure called the epiglottis. Our vocal cords in the larynx close to protect the airway, and the larynx rises under the back of the tongue just in time for our upper esophageal sphincter to open and admit the bolus or liquid.

If you place your fingers over your Adam's Apple (the laryngeal prominence of the thyroid cartilage), you may be able to feel this movement when you swallow. Try it. Fingers on the Adam's Apple, swallow, feel it rise. As the larynx moves back down, we exhale. Normally, this chain of events takes under a second. Try to swallow again with fingers on your throat. But this time, see if you can sense when you inhale, hold your breath, and exhale. Ready? Fingers on the laryngeal prominence, breath hold, swallow, movement up, and movement down as you exhale.

We learn this complex dance of coordination and timing as infants and toddlers. We maintain these oral, pharyngeal, laryngeal, esophageal and respiratory skills, unless injured. In the elderly, this fine motor coordination may begin to falter. Such breakdowns result in occasional coughing at the mild end of these deficits, but sometimes choking or aspiration happens when more severe.

We can be more deliberate about, or more mindful of, exhaling during our chewing and after we swallow, to not only increase safety, but also to take advantage of opportunities for retronasal smelling to contribute to the experience of flavor. If we chew more slowly, we can bring our attention to exhaling. Usually we don't even think about the process of eating. It's rapid and automatic. It goes by so quickly. Ever eat something so fast that you don't remember even swallowing it? The only proof you may have that you actually ate it is an empty plate or a crumbled wrapper. But fast eating makes it impossible to savor. There's little satisfaction in it, so we might overeat as if quantity can make up for lost quality. When we eat fast, we're usually distracted. We don't give our senses their due. Here's how we can!

Try to carve out a few peaceful moments to eat. Don't think about where you've been or where you have to go. Turn off the electronics. Just be present in the moment with your food or drink. Let go of everything. Gently focus on what's on your plate and in your mouth.

Leisurely mastication and breathing maximizes the experience of flavor. Taking time to mindfully eat, as well as smell, is the gateway to recovery of the senses. It is the first step to what I described as *Deep Tasting* in my previous books. Deep tasting is the key to appreciation and enjoyment. So slow down. Savor, as best you can. Breathe.

Describing this process is not meant to torment those of you suffering from smell and taste loss. Understanding is key to appreciating what's been lost, what needs rehabilitation, and how to go about it. When you cannot taste a favorite food now, some brain trickery in the form of evoking memories is worth a try. Even while we do stimulation therapy to re-establish neural connections, the Evoking Memory Exercises support our efforts when nothing is registering (anosmia) or is distastefully doing so (parosmia).

EVOKING MEMORY FOR TASTE AND FLAVOR

If you have a diminished, or loss of, perception for any of the 5-basic tastes or flavor-creating mechanisms, add the following memory-evoking exercises to daily taste/flavor therapy. It is recommended that you do these exercises twice a day. The exercises require only a teaspoon or two, so no need to worry about calories.

1. First, attempt to smell a chosen food before putting it in your mouth. Allow your sense memories and any related evoked emotions to work for you as described in the previous chapter.
2. Next, place the food in your mouth. Feel your tongue meet the item and your lips close around it. Bring your memories of texture, taste, emotions and pleasure to the act of moving the food around your mouth.
3. Take the time to leisurely chew and move the substance around to different areas of your mouth. How does that feel? Are you producing saliva? As taste or flavor may be diminished or unpleasant in the present, call up your memories of the past pleasant taste, sensations and emotions associated with the food. Superimpose those past experiences on the current act of tasting by turning up the volume of those memories to drown out the sound of any disagreeable, diminished, or missing sensations in the present. You may notice that you inhale while the food is in the front of your mouth and between your teeth, then you hold your breath when you swallow. After you swallow, exhale again. Again, use your imagination to recall taste, texture, pleasure or other emotions.

EVOKING MEMORY FOR SOMATOSENSORY LOSS

The sensory receptors and neural pathways that serve temperature, touch, pressure, and pain are proximate and run adjacent to those of basic taste. Therefore, it's entirely possible that somatosensory perception can be impaired as a result of anything that compromises the taste receptors and pathways. If so, you may not be able to feel, or not fully sense, the smoothness of cream cheese or the crunchiness of nuts, the heft of a mouthful of sandwich, the coldness of ice cream, the wetness and warmth of hot coffee, and maybe not even the pain of spicy, chili burn.

If you tested for the Somatosensory Components of Smell and Taste in Chapter Six, and found that you're experiencing a deficit in this area, try working with the following exercise. A note of warning: If you have a diminished sense of temperature or pain (burn) you need to exercise caution not to injure yourself. Test temperatures by placing a drop of the food or liquid on your wrist. If using a piquant spice like chili, use no more than a quarter teaspoon.

EVOKING SOMATOSENSORY MEMORY EXERCISE:

1. Start with a familiar food which you might have tried recently only to find that you couldn't sense its texture, temperature, mouthfeel, or spicy burn at the present time. Without placing the food in your mouth, close your eyes and recall what it used to feel like on your tongue, how it felt biting it, chewing it, and moving it around your mouth before finally swallowing it.
2. Now place a piece of the actual food in your mouth. Bring your awareness to all the same touch points you just attempted to evoke in your memory in #1. How did the imagined experience compare with the actual? Can you get clearer memories by repeating the exercise?

3. Repeat step #1. But this time, turn up the loudness level of your memory and superimpose it on the actual food in the present moment of consuming it. Try to turn up the memory so loud that you can't distinguish that which is memory from what is actually in your mouth.

Once you know how to work with the Evoking Somatosensory Memory exercise, you can, but don't have to, carve out a special time of day to do it. But if you have somatosensory deficits, at least work with these exercises once every day during a meal. Select one item on your plate to work with that represents the diminished sensory input. For example, if it's crunch, select a crunchy item. If it's temperature, work with a warm item. It is recommended that you try to use the same food item everyday for one week before switching to another.

NINE

STEALTH THERAPY AND COMPENSATORY STRATEGIES

FLAVOR ELEMENT VARIABLES

We learned that when people have impaired smell or taste, flavor can be absent, weak, or distorted. Aroma and taste can be nonexistent, minimal, off-putting, or downright unapproachable. Also, we discovered that the somatosensory pathways for touch, pressure, temperature, and pain can also be impaired. If we're fortunate, they can remain partially or fully intact. This trigeminal pathway can provide options for therapy, as well as compensatory day to day dietary problem solving. Think of the somatosensory as a kind of stealth pathway. Metaphorically, when access is blocked to a room in a building, try the crawl space or the ventilation duct.

If you skipped the self-testing in chapter six, you'll need to do that now in order to work with the content below. Provide yourself with a detailed summary of your sensory status. These results of your self-testing create a composite picture of sensory strengths and deficits. Further, once you have this snapshot summary, it reveals which perceptual pathways need rehabilitation, those that are available to assist in that healing, or suggests options to compensate when full recovery is not realistic or is still distant. To understand how we might use this information, let's begin by looking at perceptual abilities through the lens of a common snack.

THE CHIP AND DIP SNACK

Think about a tortilla chip dipped in guacamole and spicy tomato salsa, the chunky kind. I'll walk you through some sensory properties of this snack. Then you can consult the results of your self-testing to compare how you might perceive it given your current smell and taste status. Also, take a look at the components that form the somatosensory supports of flavor perception. We'll revisit these *Flavor Element Variables* a little later. Back to the tortilla chips with guacamole and salsa. Our chip and dip snack.

The tortilla chip is crunchy, toasted, sometimes smokey, and usually salty. The avocado in the guacamole has been mashed smooth and cool. In the salsa, we meet a savory umami in the tomato cubes, tender islands bobbing in a sea of spicy, acidic juice. There are crunchy, piquant onions and bitter garlic, sour lemon juice, and zesty, clingy cilantro leaves that also bring a bit of bitterness to the mix. Of course, there's that quintessential chili burn.

We can experience this complex treat in several places in the nose, mouth and throat. Maybe you can't smell the corn in the tortilla, but you might detect the toasted or smokey aspects. You might not want to take a whiff of the salsa, because the chili can make you sneeze. Instead, take a bite. The burn can start on your lips or on the tongue. Possibly, you'll feel it inside your cheeks or at the back of the throat. The bitter flashes of cilantro are picked up as a refreshing counterpoint. The tomato and lemon may cause the inside of your lips to pucker. Onion and garlic brings sweet, sour and bitter, to the burn of the chili. Sense that trio of heat rise up from the back of your tongue as you swallow.

So there you have it. A popular snack that carries so much richness, the aromas, all 5-basic tastes, and the somatosensory effects of several textures, plus pucker, and burn. Refrigerate the guacamole and salsa to add a cool temperature to the trigeminal effects. That is how someone without any impairment of smell or taste might experience it.

Assuming that you now have the results of your self-testing before you, think about how you might actually perceive our chip and dip snack, given your current perceptual status. Could you recognize what you were consuming if blindfolded? What if some of the sensory information was missing or weak but you still had other perceptions to lean on? What offending aromas might you wish to reduce or eliminate from the recipe? For example, if you are parosmic, onion or garlic can be offensive. How might you adjust the recipe? Read on for clues.

Any food or beverage can be analyzed and broken into characteristics or component parts just the way we did our chip and dip snack. So before planning a meal or treat, take out your testing summary. What do you need to avoid? What do you wish to enhance? Then consider the dish you wish to prepare. Seek information on the ingredients of those foods. Which ingredients might be a challenge or unpleasant for you? What choices can you make to compensate?

1. Consult your flavor memory. Do a little analysis just as we did with the tortilla snack. Try to remember the food aromas, flavors and textures that you were able to perceive before your sensory impairment. How might those ingredients affect you now? You may need some assistance with regard to ingredients and flavors. See #3.
2. Consult your self-test summary. Which of those aromas, flavors or textures are you unable to perceive, detect weakly, or are distorted and unpleasant? How might you compensate? What do you need to increase if weak, reduce if distorted, or replace if imperceptible or intolerable? Let's again use our chip and dip tortilla chip, avocado and salsa snack as an example.

    - Start with the tortilla chips. Not all tortilla chips are created equal. There are many different brands. If fried ones with smokey flavors attack your parosmic nose, try plain ones, or baked chips.
    - Let's move on to the onions and garlic in the salsa. If you're parosmic, these can offend you. How can you compensate? What flavor properties do the onion and garlic have? Crunch, sweet, sour (onions) bitter (garlic) and piquancy (both).

- Where can you find those components in other foods? You may have enough crunch in the tortilla chips to suit you, but you can always add chopped cilantro stems to make up for the lost onion crunch. Tiny cubes of cucumber can also add crunch. Or try chopped, fresh chili peppers for crunch and missing garlic piquancy. Cilantro leaves can add more bitterness to compensate for the garlic. One drop more of lemon juice may adjust the sour of the missing onion. If your recipe relied on onion for subtle sweetness, add just a micro-pinch of sugar.

3. Don't let this process overwhelm you. Maybe you don't have a good culinary sense of ingredients and their flavors. That's not unusual. Don't stress yourself out. Ask for help from a friend who cooks. It might be fun to sort it out together. But you can do this on your own. Consult cook books or online recipes to assist yourself in figuring out the ingredients in any dish. Once you know the ingredients, search for descriptions of their flavors. If trying to problem-solve through one recipe seems too much, forget about that particular dish. Find something that works better for you.

4. Food preparation is creative expression. Try to have fun with it. Will it take time and testing to achieve a recipe that has the right balance for you? Yes. Experiment! Don't afraid to be bold. For example, in the tortilla, guacamole and salsa snack, you may find that you want to use different varieties of tomatoes

or chilies to rebalance the recipe. Different varieties have alternative flavor profiles. You can rebalance any recipe. You may want to use atypical ingredients entirely. That's okay. Make recipes your own. This is about pleasing your own palate. You'll learn more in the section on *Flavor Element Variables*.

As a result of self-testing, you will know which aroma or flavor contributors might be missing, distorted, or available to you. Knowledge is power. When we know our status through testing, we can use what remains to help us recall and rebuild neural connections through stimulation. We can do a workaround for what is missing or unpleasant and focus on what we can perceive in order to still have an interesting, if not totally pleasing, food experience. Therefore, we can use this information both therapeutically and for daily living.

Recall that oral and nasal sensory information ends up in an area of the brain where integration with memory and emotion takes place to create the perception of flavor. But other sensory information, such as hearing and vision, also converge with these integration centers. And we already know that flavor perception is influenced and modified by visual and auditory input. Does that mean you can make food seem tastier if you put on your favorite music or serve dinner on elegant china? What if you surround yourself in a favorite color and top off the table setting with a vase of beautiful flowers? Will the food taste better? It can't hurt!

Pathways which remain intact can provide options for sensory rehabilitation. This knowledge can help you, or an SLP, decide how and which food or aromatic stimuli to use to help you learn, relearn, or compensate. Review your summary and notes from working through chapter six. What's your sensory profile? How are your somatosensory perceptions functioning? Exploiting these pathways underlies the basis for working with *Flavor Element Variables.*

INTRODUCING FLAVOR ELEMENT VARIABLES OR FEVS

Somatosensory stimuli contribute to food and drink flavor perception. We use the term *Flavor Element Variables* (*FEVs*) because they accompany smell and the basic-5 tastes to create the overall impression of flavor, and can be manipulated as variables. That is, as variables, they can be selected to be added, substituted, subtracted or eliminated from food and drink.

FEVs can assist a food's aromatic and flavor profiles, bypassing smell and taste when those perceptions are lacking, diminished, or distorted. Stimulation with these variables accompanying smell and taste can wake up the brain, assist it in eliciting memories related to flavor recognition, and create new neural connections essential to relearning. Therefore, the use of FEVs is rehabilitative. Perhaps most compelling, and of immediate benefit to people experiencing the frustration, anxiety, and distress of acute smell and taste disorders, FEVs can be used to make food more palatable. Using FEVs can greatly improve nutritional intake by increasing engagement and pleasure.

HOW TO IMPLEMENT FLAVOR ELEMENT VARIABLE (FEV) STRATEGIES

Use the FEVs to bypass, modify,or enhance smell and the basic-5 tastes. Add or substitute some of the following FEVs to foods that currently lack or distort flavor. Which FEVs might you want to include, reduce, or eliminate? Texture? Sensations? Burn? Temperature? This list gives you many options.

WHERE TO FIND FLAVOR ELEMENT VARIABLES (FEVS)?

Where do you find ideas for FEVs? Asian cookbooks are great resources for learning to add texture and piquancy (spicy heat or burn) to foods. Indian and Thai cuisines excel in piquancy, whereas Japanese cuisine can give you ideas for variation in texture and mouthfeel. Mexican cookbooks can teach you how to use chilies. But remember that food may be more tolerable served cold for patients suffering from parosmia.

Make a list of foods that you like as examples of the following textures to create a repertoire you can call upon to improve your recipes and dining experiences. Some choices can be used in preparation and cooking while others can be added impromptu, when served. An example is salt. Some cooks prefer to incorporate it into a recipe while others leave it to each individual to salt their meal as their taste dictates.

Texture variables: smooth, creamy, crunchy, sticky, airy, slippery, oily

smooth-butter or cream, cocoa butter, avocado

creamy-pudding, yogurt, ice cream, bisque

crunchy-slivers of almond or chopped nuts, ice

sticky-peanut butter, taffy, caramel, hard candy

airy-whipped potato, mousse, or meringue

slippery-egg white as in egg drop soup, wet noodles, steamed seaweed (Nori), smoked salmon or pickled fish served cold.

oily- fats and vegetable oils, foods that break down into oils

Sensation variables: carbonated or bubbly, piquant/spicy, burning, tingly or numbing, astringent or puckering

- Carbonated

  Add carbonated seltzer (0mg sodium) to juice. Try sparkling ciders and wines.

- Piquant/Spicy/Burning

  Capsaicin chilies come in a wide variety. Note that not all are hot or piquant. Piquancy is desirable for our purposes. Cayenne is more translucent whereas Habanero brings some earthy tomato paste and umami flavors. Experiment with chilies to find which are most compatible with any particularly dish. A variety of whole dried chilies can be purchased from Mexican and gourmet specialty stores. Feed individual chilies into a spice grinder. Reduce to ground powder to sample their flavor characteristics. Be careful working with chilies not to burn your eyes or nose with the ground dust. Work with a mask, eye protection and gloves. Avoid inhaling the chili dust. Remove the powder from your hands and avoid touching your eyes or mucous membranes. Remember that chilies can be weaponized, as in *pepper spray*!

If pizza is a favorite, sprinkle with chili flakes before heating, but serve cold. Choose a favorite crust texture, one that is thin and crispy, or more chewy and doughy. Parosmics may prefer to avoid garlic.

In addition to capsicum chilies, spicy heat can be found in fresh or pickled ginger, cumin and fenugreek. In some ingredients *burn* seems confined to the tongue and inner cheeks while other types, including wasabi and fresh horseradish, seem to radiate to the nose.

- Tingle/Numbness

  Sichuan "peppers" are not actually capsicum chilies. In addition to a chili-type burn, Sichuans cause lips and tongue to tingle or numb. Their varied pepper colors have their own subtle flavors which may not be detectable beyond the sensations.

- Astringency

  Drying and puckering sensations are found in sour foods, such as lemons, grapefruit, sour pickles, sauerkraut, vinegars, and foods rich in tannins, such as dark chocolate/cocoa, coffee, black or green tea, red wine, and unripened fruit, including persimmon.

Some of these foods are more astringent than others, so experiment. They tend to be high in acidity, so a word of caution. Acidity can wear on tooth enamel. Therefore, the acid should not be allowed to sit on the teeth, and it is advisable to rinse the mouth with milk and/or water as soon as possible. There are over-the-counter preparations, such as Sensodyn Pronamel® paste and mouthwash, which claim to protect the teeth against acid erosion. The use of a straw and high calcium foods, such as yogurt or ice cream, also has some protective properties.

Temperatures Variables:

Heat causes smell molecules to become volatile, increasing the aromatic potential to offend the parosmic nose. Cooler versions of many foods are easier for people with parosmia to tolerate. Experiment to see whether an altered temperature version of a favorite food or drink with which you are currently struggling can make it more tolerable, even appetizing. Try the following substitutions for their hot counterparts.

Iced- iced coffee or iced hot chocolate
Cold-room temperature bread instead of toast

cold cereal instead instead of steamy oatmeal

cold, hard boiled egg instead of scrambled or fried

shredded cold chicken salad or cold deli meats instead of freshly grilled or roasted meats

add refreshing mint, cool cucumber, yogurt, chilled condensed milk or cream

turn hot vegetables into salads by tossing with olive oil, serve cold

potatoes and root vegetables cut, cook, toss in mayonnaise or olive oil, serve cold

If a smell or flavor disorder has caused you to lose weight, and glucose intake isn't an issue, keep your calories up by adding a tolerable flavor of ice cream to crunchy nuts or chewy fruit.

Complexity and Contrasts:

To make meals interesting, create complexity by using contrasts, such as sweet/sour, sweet/salty, and smooth/crunchy. Add sour lemon or grapefruit zest and/or butter or olive oil to bitter greens, such as broccoli, Brussel sprouts, endive, or arugula. Add crunchy nuts, almond slivers, and pumpkin or sesame seeds to enliven salads and casseroles. Sprinkle lightly with a piquant spice.

FOODS TO AVOID WITH PAROSMIA

Certain foods are particularly problematic for those experiencing the distortion of aroma and flavor perception called parosmia. Troublesome items include coffee, chocolate, eggs, onions, and garlic. Meat, even toast, can be unappetizing when cooking and served hot. People complain that foods produced by searing, roasting, grilling or toasting, processes that create aromas and flavors by the Maillard Reaction or caramelization, can smell spoiled, like ashes, sewage, even excrement. People with parosmia can find these aromas nauseating. If the odors induce actual vomiting, it is best to avoid the source initially and, when able, to approach the irritant briefly and systematically to desensitize yourself to them. Take tiny whiffs. It is possible to adapt to the unpleasant source with limited exposure and by building up a tolerance.

As mentioned in our discussion of the FEVs, to avoid unpleasant dining experiences, many with parosmia gravitate toward cold and bland foods. That's a good way to ensure you get your basic nutrition covered. But it's also important to confront the disagreeable therapeutically with pleasant taste and smell memories to re-establish neural connections during the healing process. When approaching foods that seem disgusting to varying degrees, try to pull up the good memories and superimpose them over the current perceptual experience. Go back to the Evoking Memory exercises for smell and taste. Start out by approaching the offenders when they are cold. Wade in slowly and briefly over time, remembering what they used to smell and taste like and any pleasant emotions associated with those foods. Eventually, you may be able to eat them with less distress. While trying to keep your nutrition and weight up, FEVs can distract from some unpleasant smells and tastes. Also add FEVs to enhance the meal.

Aromas and flavors are made up of complex molecular components. Parosmia can function like a filter that lets only the nasty components pass through. Recognize that your senses are only giving you partial or distorted information. Try to use your imagination to recreate the whole. Keep that at the forefront of your mind while approaching aromas and tastes that currently seem repugnant. Remember that you need to retrieve memories to complete the picture of what that food once smelled and tasted like.

TEN

REGAINING STRENGTH

Our mouths and noses, the first way stations to processing smell and taste, are not disconnected from the rest of the body, but are integrated with the respiratory system. Just as we train to regain smell and taste, patients sometimes need to strengthen muscles for chewing, swallowing, and respiration. When we talk about strengthening muscles, the approach we take depends on the cause of the dysfunction. Some disabilities that affect the autonomic nervous system, including COVID, require a slow, calibrated method that avoids exertion and emphasizes resting and recovery time.

Since July 2021, the CDC has made available a list of Long COVID symptoms for health providers on the CDC.gov website. Many would do good to read it. One of the hallmarks of PACS is Post-Exertional Malais or PEM. It is a condition with a disheartening and frustrating dynamic. The CDC describes PEM this way.

"Post-exertional malaise (PEM) is the worsening of symptoms following even minor physical or mental exertion, with symptoms typically worsening 12 to 48 hours after activity and lasting for days or even weeks."

In other words, patients try the usual route of recovery. They push themselves, sometimes only a little, then they crash. And the regression can last for days, even weeks, as the quote above from the CDC describes. The process of resuming normal activity and exercise is the opposite of that which is recommended in training and physical therapy. Many doctors still do not understand this and think the patient is malingering. They will advise the patient to just get on with things, but this is to their detriment. Most physicians and physical therapists encourage the patient to press on, to push to increase endurance and strength. That was how these professionals were trained to think, and that's the traditional approach to rehabilitation. But for someone with Long COVID or dysautonomia, pushing can lead to a collapse. The professionals needs to consider the individual before them, engage in some creative rethinking and adapt their methodology. I would refer these professionals to the work of David Putrino who recently has advanced guidelines for how to differentiate and treat these patients.

Some Long Haulers, many who have been runners, say that when they've tried to return to aerobic exercise too soon after the acute phase of COVID (approximately 4-6 weeks) it started them on a downward spiral. Those knowledgable about recovery say only the gentlest of activities should be attempted for 12 weeks after COVID. Instead of long walks or any kind of aerobics, light weight training and toning is advised. Also gentle yoga is recommended. Stress of any kind needs to be minimized. Therefore, meditation may be helpful. Once established that a patient is actually experiencing Long COVID, these guidelines are particularly true.

Again, the usual coaching to motivate and encourage the athlete to excel is counterproductive for PACS patients. They cannot be pushed to the limit without triggering flare ups and self-defeating set backs. Any physician or other caregiver who pushes the patient to work harder to get back to normal, does not understand the nature of Long COVID. These patients are contending with vascular disease, inflammation, autoimmune and autonomic nervous system disorders, just for starters. Physicians need to read the CDC website papers on Long COVID because these facts have been known for quite some time.

So it's important to keep this warning in mind while working on any exercises in this chapter. The exercises here are meant to help patients get started. The professional who can help fine tune an exercise program for chewing, swallowing, speech or voice is a speech-language pathologist who has hopefully educated themselves about Long COVID. If the exercises here don't seem to apply to you, skip them. If they seem too difficult, reach out to an SLP through the American Speech-Language-Hearing Association (see Resource section).

It's tricky to perform an exercise straight from a book. An SLP will be able to interpret and adapt an exercise to your personal needs, but they must understand your specific physical challenges. Make sure they are familiar with the pacing issues for dysautonomia and Long COVID so they don't push you too hard. As a patient, don't be afraid to speak up. Advocate for yourself. Carry print-outs of literature about Long COVID as you may need to educate people, even professionals. A doctor or therapist who isn't open-minded and doesn't have the humility to learn, even from a patient, can be dangerous.

EXERCISES FOR CHEWING AND SWALLOWING

Just as you might work with a physical therapist to gain strength in your torso and limb muscles, your best guide to recovering strength in chewing and swallowing muscles is the speech-language pathologist, particularly one who is board certified in dysphagia. Some of the exercises described below will be familiar to the SLP. Again, if you are an SLP, take your cue from the patient. Do not urge them to exert themselves. Minimal effort.

A mirror is needed for several of these exercises.

SMELLING MUSCLES? YES!

We are so accustomed to thinking of smell in a passive way that we may not realize the taking of deep whiffs usually stimulates the contraction of muscles around the nostrils, enabling them to flare or sometimes to wrinkle up our noses. Try the following exercises. Do not feel you must do them one after another in one session.

- Nose flaring: While looking in a mirror, take a breath in through your nose and dilate your nostrils to open them. Do this 3 times on 3 inhalations. Ready? Inhale on a flare, exhale. Two more times. Rest.

- Nose wrinkling: Sometimes we wrinkle our noses up like a bunny to express displeasure. But the bunny does it to inhale and smell. Wrinkle your nose up 3 times, once on each of 3 inhalations. So, inhale, wrinkle, exhale. Repeat twice more. Rest.

UVULA AND SOFT PALATE

Look in a mirror, open your mouth and shine a flashlight inside toward the back. You will see a bit of tissue hanging down in a slight v shape that forms arches on both sides. This hanging thing is called the uvula, and it is part of the soft palate. When we swallow, the ability to raise the soft palate forms a seal to prevent liquid and food particles from being snorted out the nose. The closure of the soft palate also contributes to a shift in air pressure in the oropharynx that assists in swallowing, and it prevents a hypernasal sounding voice quality. While looking in the mirror, try to raise the uvula. As it rises, note the arches on both sides of the uvula smooth out as they straighten up.

- Think of a high vocal pitch and see if you can raise the uvula. Doing your best imitation of a soprano's high note. Ready? Sing "Ah, ah, ah." Rest. Do this 2 more times. Then rest.
- Yawn. Open your mouth, think how you feel when you're fighting off sleepiness, and do a big yawn. Usu-

ally, just starting to yawn causes a full, automatic one to ensue. Do it twice, then rest.

LIPS MUSCLES

We need strong muscles around our lips to be able to purse and smile. These muscles not only enable us to kiss and express emotions, they also help us keep the liquids from leaking out our mouths so we can drink froma cup and take food off a spoon or fork. In addition, the lips form an anterior seal or valve that can assist the tongue muscles in adjusting the intraoral pressure necessary to swallow.

- While looking in a mirror, smile as broadly as you can, then pucker up your lips as if to kiss, ending on a kiss noise. Do it 3 times, then rest.

TONGUE MUSCLES

- Stick your tongue out as if to lick food off your lips. Sweep you tongue around in a circular motion. Lick the top lip in a clockwise motion from left upper corner to right corner. Then lick your bottom lip clockwise from lower right corner to lower left corner, making one big circular clockwise sweep. Rest. Repeat, but his time do it in reverse, lick counterclockwise on the top lip, then counterclockwise on the lower lip, making one big counterclockwise sweep. Rest.

INSIDE YOUR MOUTH

The following sweeping movements of your tongue are useful in dislodging food residue from your mouth. Think about peanut butter or mashed potatoes remaining on your teeth, gums, or inside your cheeks after eating. What did you do in the past? In addition to sipping water? Right! You probably used your tongue to remove the food.

- Lick the inside of your lips from left to right, then right to left. Reverse. Rest. Lick the full arch of your upper teeth from side to side. Outer side and inner side of the teeth. Now bottom arch, from side to side. Rest.
- Run you tongue across the inside of your cheeks. Both sides. Then rest.

CHEWING MUSCLES:

- Pretend you're chewing gum. Make 3 small, circular chewing movements with your lips closed. Reverse direction. Make 3 small, circular chewing movements. Rest. Keeping the movements tiny and gentle is particularly important if you've had past problems with the jaw or TMJ, the temporomandibular joint. Instead of circular movements, a simple, straight up and down chewing motion may be preferable for those with past TMJ issues. Please use your judgment.

TONGUE AND SWALLOW MUSCLES:

This exercise actually has a name. It's called the Masako or Tongue Hold Maneuver. It can strengthen muscles that prevent aspiration.

- Stick your tongue forward between your teeth. Gently bite down on the tip of your tongue. Swallow dry (Only saliva. No food.) Release by pulling your tongue back into your mouth. Rest. Repeat.

VOICE AND LARYNGEAL MUSCLES

Here are some simple exercises to help in recovery of the strength and flexibility of the laryngeal muscles essential to protecting the airway and producing voice.

- Push the palms of your hands together and gently say "ah" in one long sustained sound for two-seconds. Rest. Repeat. Work towards a voice quality that is not breathy and sounds clear.
- Covering your mouth with a tissue, cough once sharply with a good solid voice. Rest. Repeat.
- With gentle loudness, lips closed, hum from a low pitch to a high pitch on one continuous "mmmm" up and "mmmm" down. Rest Repeat.

BREATHING

Breathing is a natural act until it isn't. And there is no smelling, and no detection of flavor without breathing. Disruptions and deviations of breathing can begin at birth or at any time thereafter. Irregular breathing patterns are an adaptation to illness, injury, or trauma, that may become habitual, persisting long after the original cause has resolved.

During respiratory illness, when our noses or lungs are congested, we can struggle to inhale any way possible. Breathing can be shallow, and we might gasp or use our upper chest and shoulder muscles to expand the lungs. Recurrent problems with allergies, sinus problems, or asthma can force us to alter natural patterns. Structural injury to our noses, ribs, back and spine, and to some degree, disorders of the upper gastrointestinal tract, can disrupt normal breathing patterns, forcing us to deviate, at least, in the short term. Often these patterns can carry over into long-term maladaptations. When we recover, we may not realize we've habituated aberrant patterns.

Post-traumatic stress, as well as anxiety and depression, can alter normal breathing patterns. If we live in a state of stress, we may clench muscles of the jaw, shoulders, arms. We may hold our breath at times. When we are in fight or flight mode, respiration rates increase, blood flow shifts to tensed muscles of legs, heart, torso and lungs, and away from the digestive tract. People may also seek to suppress emotions after terrible shock or loss through tensing muscles and holding their breath. All of these conditions can contribute to the habituation of inefficient breathing patterns in need of retraining.

Since so many cases of smell disorders occur with respiratory illness or injury, particularly with severe COVID when people may have been on ventilators or auxiliary sources of oxygen during and after recovery, it's important to check on our breathing patterns. We've also discussed how swallowing disorders, regardless of cause, can involve poor coordination of breathing with swallowing. When timing and coordination of breathing and swallowing are out of phase, we need to become conscious of the pattern and take steps to correct it by learning to be deliberate about breathing, holding our breath, swallowing, and releasing the breath.

To summarize. It's important to: 1. Become conscious of breathing patterns and identify any irregularities. 2. If necessary, restore efficient and healthy breathing patterns. 3. To be able to control the breathing process in a compensatory manner when neuromuscular disorders, particularly progressive ones, make restoration of normal patterns unlikely, and when there is discoordination of swallowing and breathing.

In the next exercises, you will explore these questions about your respiration and breathing patterns.

- How do you currently breathe?
- What muscular patterns do you use?
- What are efficient, healthy breathing patterns?
- Are you able to hold and control your breath?
- Are your muscles strong enough? At least minimal strength is essential for healthy breathing, as well as safe eating, swallowing, and flavor perception.

DISCOVER YOUR CURRENT BREATHING PATTERN.

Sit upright on a firm chair. It may be useful to move a chair in front of a full length mirror to see, as well as feel, what your body is doing. But first try detecting your breathing pattern just by feeling. If you have trouble sitting, you can do the exercise lying on your back, face up, head straight, legs parallel and uncrossed.

Place one hand on your collar bone and the other further down, just above your navel in the space between your lower ribs. This is the area of the diaphragm, although that is inside the ribs, and what you actually feel are abdominal muscles. Don't try to do anything but observe which hand rises as you are breathing, and answer these questions.

1. Is your hand sensing movement in your upper chest? Are you holding or raising your shoulders as you breathe? If so, you are using accessory muscles to compensate. It may be, or has been, necessary for you at some time for some reason. We can see runners briefly use these muscles to recover in moments after a peak effort. That is normal. It is also a pattern that can be seen in asthmatics. But this is not a normal pattern in the sense of being efficient in healthy persons. It is a pattern seen in those struggling to breathe.
2. If you're not feeling the pattern described in #1, good. Then, is your bottom hand, the one just above the navel, being pushed outward as you inhale and back in as you exhale? That's a healthy, efficient pattern.

Without trying to do anything, keep your hands positioned, breathe for a few moments, and just notice which parts of your torso are moving your hands. Okay, got your current pattern?

Let's make sure you're not experiencing any extraneous tension.

- This time, as you observe your breathing, you can deliberately release any tension. Say "s-s-s-s," without stopping as you exhale and release any tension around your neck and shoulders. Let the shoulders drop. Did you feel any tension in your neck and shoulders release? You may have noticed, that as soon as you reach the very end of the "s-s-s," that you automatically inhale. You didn't have to *try* to inhale, it just happened. It's a natural, automatic reaction.
- Try saying the "s-s-s" again, this time as you near the end of the sound, make the conscious choice to close your mouth and inhale through the nose.

What is one breathing cycle?

Exhaling on s-s-s, followed by a quick, automatic inhalation through the nose was one breath cycle. Of course, it can be done without the s-s-s. We were just using the s-s-s sound so you could hear that your exhalation was unbroken and continuous. It's a way of checking that you weren't holding or stopping the breath. Now, allow yourself to just breathe through the nose quietly, feeling yourself exhaling and inhaling for a few restful cycles.

Prolonging the s-s-s nonstop, as long as you can, maybe 15-20 seconds, pushes the respiratory muscles to work hard.

It's helpful in clearing the lungs. You can try that if you ever feel congested. Was the s-s-s continuous? You're not holding your breath? If you happen to detect that you're holding your breath, you've learned something valuable about how your body functions. Note that if you are congested and you do the breathing exercise with the s-s-s, it can trigger coughing. If it's just a few gentle coughs, fine. But a coughing fit can be exhausting, and it can irritate the larynx. You may not feel physically up to a coughing fit. You must decide whether you want to risk triggering one or not. And if you've learned what constitutes one breath cycle, you do not need to use the s-s-s for further breath work here.

The yogic traditions have handed down ways to strengthen the respiratory system that can help during and after recovery from disease. Yogic breathing is calming, can improve blood chemistry and lower blood pressure. Although yoga, as well as meditation, has been appropriated in the West and is often marketed divorced from its Eastern spiritual roots, medical practitioners have found these techniques proven ways to de-stress and promote health. One organization working with health-enhancing breath work is Stasis.life which offers online videos and tutorials. See Resources section.

Let's practice silent, restful breathing (without the s-s-s-sound). This is *efficient, healthy breathing.*

- Place one hand on either left or right side of your lowest ribs. Place the other hand just above the navel again, on the space between your lowest left and right ribs. Take a slow, gentle breath in through your nostrils to the silent count of 3. And as you do, feel your lower ribs slightly move out laterally, and the space between the ribs above the navel push your hand outward. Then observe the movements reverse as you exhale to the silent count of 3. These will be small movements. You should not be forcing or efforting.

- This is resting, intercostal-diaphragmatic breathing. It is an efficient and healthy pattern. It is what you should be doing, without counting, of course, whenever you're just sitting or lying down.

BUILDING CAPACITY AND STRENGTH

To build up lung capacity and supporting muscular strength, you can increase your silent count. Inhale to 4 and exhale to 6. Don't force it. Do what you can comfortably. If you can only make the count to 3 or 4 that's fine to begin. Be aware of continuous exhalation without stops. To avoid hyperventilating as a beginner, rest after each cycle for about 30 seconds. Repeat. Rest. Do that 3 times, if you can. Do not push yourself. If it was easy for you, work up to 5 repetitions, later 10 repetitions. If you have Long COVID or dysautonomia, do less.

Over the next weeks, reduce the resting time between the cycles from 30 seconds to only 15 seconds, then 5 seconds. When you can do 5 cycles inhaling to the silent count of 4 and exhaling to 6 or 8, without feeling dizzy or light headed, or triggering any panic attacks, then you can drop the 5 second rest periods between the cycles and go for 10 repetitions. There's no reason to push yourself. Do the amount that is comfortable for you. If you have Long COVID or dysautonomia, do less.

BREATH HOLDING

Various therapeutic swallowing procedures employed by speech-language pathologists use breath-holding techniques to close the vocal folds of the larynx so that aspiration of foods is avoided; that is, so food particles and liquids do not go down the trachea (the "wrong pipe"). But the larynx is not a one-way street. It's not just a matter of what can go down.

When the vocal folds are closed, air cannot pass upward from the lungs to the trachea, then out through the larynx at the top of the trachea. From there air is usually expelled by mouth, or if the mouth is closed, up through the nose. But none of this happens when the vocal folds are closed as we are holding our breath. Most of us learn how to hold our breath when we are still children, but how can we be sure that we are successfully stopping our breath? Here are a few ways:

1. *Holding the breath when breathing through the mouth*

   Say "uh" as in the word "up." Begin the uh as if to sustain the sound, then cut it off by holding the breath. You may detect a movement in your throat, the shutting of the vocal folds. And the sound should stop.

   - Try it again, this time hold you hand over your open mouth. Position your hand in front of your mouth, open your mouth and start saying "uh."

Feel your breath? Now, hold your breath. Can you feel that no breath is coming out of your mouth?

- Were you able to stop the breath? If not, this can mean that you just need practice. But it can also mean that your laryngeal muscles need strengthening. You may find confirmation of laryngeal weakness if you also experience shortness of breath as you go about your daily activities.

Let's try the breath holding again.

- This time, start the "uh" and gently press your palms together. That should stop the sound momentarily.
- Another way to experience the stopping or holding of the breath is to start the uh, then try to grunt, *gently* pressing down, as if moving your bowels. Executing this exercise with more effort is called the Valsalva maneuver. However, repeatedly grunting hard can lead to laryngeal injury in people with normal strength. So easy does it!

The object of including this exercise here is just to give you a simple feeling of how to stop or hold the breath. You may wish to work under the guidance of a speech-language pathologist if you're having swallowing or choking issues. Of course, if the swallowing or choking problem is recent, you should get a medical evaluation, and possibly a referral for a swallow study.

2. *Holding the breath while breathing through the nose*

Begin with two cycles of restful, efficient breathing through the nose while you hold your hand under your nostrils to feel the breath coming out as you exhale. After inhaling for the third cycle, stop your breath. You should not feel any breath on your hand. Hold to a silent count of 3, then exhale. You should again feel the breath on your hand.

People who have suffered respiratory illnesses, and those who have required breathing support will likely need to strengthen their laryngeal and inspiratory/expiratory muscles. It's all a matter of degree, and according to individual needs. The exercises can be fine-tuned by a clinician.

RESPIRATORY TRAINING AIDS

Often patients in hospitals will encounter, or be sent home with, simple devices designed for improving respiration. But if you weren't hospitalized, never received respiratory therapy, or never thought you needed or wanted to do it, there are many types of breathing exercise aids you can investigate now.

A fun way to begin to develop breath control and respiratory endurance is by playing woodwind-type instruments, such as various types of plastic flutes, kazoos, and harmonicas, most of which can be acquired inexpensively at toy stores or online.

There are training devices to develop Expiratory Muscle Strength Training (EMST), such as The Breather®, The EMST150®, and The Expand-a-Lung®. See the Resources section of this book. Affordable and designed as rehabilitation devices, their use can improve swallowing and laryngeal function. They are also used for training by singers and athletes. The resistance levels are adjustable according to the individual's strength and needs. However, they may not be appropriate for someone experiencing PEM. Professional guidance is advisable.

APPENDIX

EXTENDING SCOPE OF PRACTICE

Speech-language pathologists are needed to play a role in the rehabilitation of smell and taste. SLPs who are already working with dysphagia are best positioned skill-wise of any allied medical professionals to become specialists in smell and taste rehabilitation. The expertise you have already begun to acquire in this book should be considered related to, or a subspecialty within, the dysphagia area.

What else will you need to be able to function competently in this new subspecialty? You will need to understand flavor. You will need to be able to manipulate the elements of flavor. Much of this knowledge will start with visceral memory. You just need to tap into it. You will be greatly aided by becoming a serious amateur in tasting. Don't be intimidated. Most professional tasters have solid but average palates, not the rarest of talents. It takes exposure, discipline, motivation. Passion helps. Tasting is a skill. But it's great fun and life-enriching. We largely acquire tasting skills through guidance and experience. See Poupon et al. 2019. You can read about the process of becoming a sommelier by checking out Bosker's amusing 2017 book, also in the References section. Here's my advice. Select a food or drink that you greatly appreciate which has a tradition of tasting, such as wine, chocolate, beer, or cheese. If you're a serious cook, that can also jump-start your tasting education. Take classes. Find a mentor.

We've made a start in this book on the basics for a new specialty. But dig deeper. There's much ongoing research that is highly technical and assumes backgrounds in chemistry, biology, and neurology. SLPs are professionals, so you will acquire any skills you may need to further advance. I'm an elderly person now; my horizons are limited. I may kick-start this subspecialty, but you will guide it into the future.

In this Appendix, you will find additional information to supplement what you've already learned in the earlier sections of this book. Here you'll read an overview of the basic neurology of the olfactory and gustatory systems, but not the details of neurochemistry or biology. That is not essential for our immediate purposes. My goal in this book is more practical than theoretical. I hope you will go on to do research in this field, but my immediate concern is that we get clinicians on their feet as quickly as possible, ready to respond to patients in need.

In addition to the self-tests in the patient-centered chapters of the book, SLPs will find lists of standardized, formal tests in the Resources section. Formal testing may become necessary if you need to submit qualitative assessments and quantitative data for the record and third party payments. I hope you will push Medicare, Medicaid, and private insurers to cover therapy for smell and taste disorders. It's not easy to create new precedents. We can get patients diagnosed. We can make a case for those suffering from Long COVID-related smell and taste disorders under the Americans for Disability Act for chefs and food writers, but others, not so much. Partner with ENTs, band together with colleagues. Make your case to ASHA. Welcome to the frontier!

Again, I want to stress how much you are needed. Involvement in COVID-related sensory disabilities is just the tip of the iceberg. COVID is not the first virus to affect the chemical senses, and it won't be the last. As you have read, there are many other non-viral causes of smell and taste loss. Among the most common is aging. Normal aging. So I'd like to direct your attention to this neglected area.

Think about the elderly, those over 70, who may be losing weight. Look beyond their other presenting disabilities. Something additional may be going unnoticed. If the physician has ruled out disease, our training leads us to first suspect poor dentition or swallowing problems. But let's also start thinking about how over the years, the foods that older people used to like have slowly lost appeal. It's possible these patients can hardly smell it. Food flavor may seem so bland now, the elderly may start avoiding it. There's no motivation to eat. Voila! Weight loss. Nutritional deficiencies. Accelerating health decline gets filed under, "she was just old." Well, maybe not. Maybe the rapid decline was preventable.

Another case to consider. Maybe an elderly person has been gaining weight, begins to spike their blood pressure, or is suddenly a borderline diabetic. The first thing the doctor is going to do is try BP meds. Our primary care physicians don't have much time with patients these days, and many are not asking enough questions. It's likely they will shove a prescription diet at the patient. Consider that maybe it's not *what* the patient is eating, but *how* they are preparing it. Are they compensating for a lack of flavor by increasing sugar or salt? Are they selecting foods that are saltier or sweeter? Why? Probably, it's to compensate for decreased flavor perception!

If we want people to decrease their intake of sugar or sodium, we need to know their smell and taste status. We need to test their perception. Remember that flavor = smell + the 5-basic tastes + the trigeminal aspects. Any diminution in perception of any of those components of flavor can lead people to rebalance their intake to compensate. We are flavor-driven creatures!

Failing to consider sensory loss, weakness, or distortion as a contributor to poor nutrition is a set-up for long-term noncompliance with respect to any prescribed diet. SLPs can work with dietitians to optimize sensory perception through the compensatory Flavor Element Variables (FEVs). Dietitians think about calories, nutrients and textures. They need the SLP who understands smell, taste, and flavor as a partner. Possibly, using the compensatory FEVs may mean the patient doesn't have to change their diet much at all, but simply drop the added sugar or salt. But they can be persuaded to do so only is there are other paths to flavor.

It's easy to attribute poor nutrition in the elderly to they're being "finicky" or as a symptom of mental decline. Maybe some of the deterioration is a result of *flavor* decline. Don't settle for a pat explanation without doing the diagnostic examination. It's no better than a physician shrugging off someone's complaints about fatigue as a lack of sleep without checking their blood work.

SLPs are already serving many nursing facility residents for neurological disorders, including dysphagia. Part of your exam should explore smell and taste. We can be providing more than input on texture. We can work more effectively with physicians, dietitians and caregivers. We want to motivate dysphagia patients by introducing appetizing aromas and flavors. Give them a reason to want to open their mouths!

MOTIVATION

Clinical education and practice stress the mechanics of enabling patients to perform skills that are quantifiable and measurable. We don't often ask about motivation. We need to think about it. Seriously. Ask the right questions. Why would a patient want to avoid a particular food or drink? Focused on the ability to chew and swallow, SLPs might not ask whether a "fussy" eater can properly smell or taste. Even worse, whether the food the patient is offered smells or tastes disgusting to them, as often is the case in parosmia. Investigate! Medications. Post-viral illness. Chemotherapy. Radiation. Head trauma. Immediately your alarm should go off. Think about the possibility that the patient, particularly one who has a history of illness, is experiencing the result of degenerating neural connections or new faulty ones established during recovery. What if they can't taste anything, or hardly at all? What if that which they were being fed was absolutely nauseating to them? The only way to know is to test.

Particularly in the case of children, we need to consider the possibility of conditioned food aversions which occur when a new food is introduced at a time when the child is experiencing unpleasant symptoms from a concurrent illness. A gastrointestinal bug, perhaps. Maybe they vomited their lunch, which just happened to include an unfamiliar food. Or possibly something emotionally distressing happened when a new food was introduced. Trauma can be encoded in their sensory memory along with the new food.

Conditioning can be recognized through questioning the child's caregiver about the time the food was first introduced. Was the child ill or in an agitated state when the food was first encountered? What exactly were the physical and environmental conditions when the food was first offered? Was the family in crisis, having lots of arguments at meal time? When you have a picture of what was going on when the food was introduced, then turn you attention to the rejected food itself.

Is the problem not specific to one particular food? Is there an aversion or avoidance of all foods that have the same texture, for example? Does everything crunchy cause the child to cringe? Or does the food have components that are of one particular basic taste, sour or umami, for example? Do your best cranial nerve examination, including all the sensory testing for touch, the basic-5 tastes, and smell. Then analyze the food that is being rejected for its flavor components.

A skilled clinician can reintroduce important cultural or family foods through various techniques of distraction and deconditioning. Change the flavor, change the texture, change the presentation, then slowly withdraw them to mirror the way the food is traditionally served. This can take months! There are ways to do this when absolutely necessary, for example, when a particular food is truly indispensable to a culture. But sometimes these attempts should be deferred until the child is older, can understand and choose to cooperate.

Pediatric SLPs may have a degree of familiarity with developmentally challenged children who are considered "picky-eaters." Sorry, but that is not a clinical description. It is imprecise, and it is, albeit unintentionally, disparaging, in my opinion. The characterization does not consider the innate wisdom residing in even disabled bodies, and it underestimates the evolutionary significance of finding foods acceptable to the nose and palate. If motor pathways are injured, why not consider that the sensory pathways are also? When a child wrinkles their nose, turns their head or pushes their food away, they are communicating. We need to better read these signals. Something is offensive to them. Their idiosyncratic, perceptual wiring may be telling them that the food tastes like something rancid or toxic, something disgusting and unacceptable. Respect the child's innate human intelligence.

How can we enable a child to discover that which is offered is acceptable, even interesting or pleasing? If that's even wise or possible. Too often, because it seems most practical, we target the specific foods and simply eliminate them or do workarounds. But consider what it is about those foods that are so offensive. We can do a better job of analyzing the specific aspects of smell, taste, and the trigeminal components, as well as consider the possibility of conditioning. I hope this book will enable you to problem solve in new ways.

The motivation to eat is important, and not just for children. The consequences of devaluing food preferences is weight loss, compensatory weight gain, and certainly compromised nutrition and health. Unpleasant distortions of smell and taste are serious threats to well-being. We must begin by attributing an underlying reason to even our most intellectually challenged patients, and engage in hypothesis testing about how they may be perceiving the smell and taste of their foods. When you have a complete picture, regardless of the patient's age or etiology, you can decide whether the course of rehabilitation should emphasize deconditioning for aversion, desensitization, sensory training or compensatory alternatives. When SLPs understand as much about smell and taste as they do about chewing and swallowing, we will raise the bar in clinical treatment.

AN OVERVIEW OF SMELL AND TASTE PERCEPTION

You will find a relevant, rather than detailed, discussion of olfactory and gustatory physiology here in this Appendix. The purpose here is to facilitate an understanding of how to think about therapeutic intervention, and not to prepare you for a medical school examination. If you want to review anatomy and physiology, as well as the perception of smell and taste, from the cellular to the cognitive levels, I recommend beginning with the sources listed on the opposite page. Also check out the References section of this book.

Basic anatomical diagrams of the olfactory and gustatory neural pathways can be found here:

https://brain-for-ai.fandom.com/wiki/Olfactory_pathway?-file=Olfaction.png

and here

https://brain-for-ai.fandom.com/wiki/Olfactory_pathway?-file=Gustatory_pathway.png

To go deeper, there are highly informative anatomy and physiology videos on YouTube, including those by Ninja Nerd and Kevin Tokoph's Catalyst University. Look for medical school faculty presenters. Check the credentials of the presenters. Many searchable sources detail the neural pathways, the neurochemistry involved in converting odorant and taste molecules into neurotransmitters, and describe the basic decoding and organization of the olfactory bulbs and the tastebud receptors. I've found the three dimensional aspects of these video presentations to be more helpful than textbooks. And you'll be in good company. Subscribers to these sites appear to include medical students. Also, because books take so long to produce, they may not reflect groundbreaking research in olfaction and gustation which is still unfolding as you read this. Of course, you should not stop with videos and online content. Use the topics contained in videos to do searches for original research.

Here are overviews of some essential points for our purposes.

SMELL PERCEPTION

The perception of smell begins when odor molecules are inhaled, whether passively or intentionally sniffed. The molecules travel up the nasal passages and are picked up by the cilia of receptor cells in the mucosal epithelium. Mucus in the nose, and saliva in the mouth, are essential to the breakdown and uptake of these odorant and taste molecules. So consider the effects of dryness or overproduction of these fluids.

In the receptor cells, the odorant molecules cause chemical reactions which generate action potentials. Of all our senses, Cranial Nerve 1, the Olfactory Nerve, is the body's most direct, single-synaptic route to the brain, crossing from the nerve endings in the nasal epithelium through the Cribriform Plate of the Ethmoid bone to the Olfactory Bulb. The neurotransmitters present there in such a way that they are taken up by specialized mitral cells in the Glomeruli. This begins the recognition and encoding process before further referral along the olfactory tract to nuclei specializing in memory and emotion. Smell can evoke episodic, emotional memories. But more often, smell evokes pure sense memories. Note that some neurochemical processes are inhibitory, so only the most excitatory odorants get through. And there is also adaptation or sensory fatigue, so that detection can be decreased. *These effects can have a direct bearing on the choice and manner of presentation of stimuli in therapy or training.*

TASTE/FLAVOR

Smell stimulates salivation, preparing our mouths to receive food. Once food is in our mouths, as we chew and exhale, as saliva manipulates and makes molecular compounds available for uptake, retronasal smells are generated up the nasopharynx and are picked up by the olfactory receptor cells embedded in the oral and pharyngeal mucosal lining, as well as in the epiglottal and esophageal areas. The retronasal smells combine with the basic-5 tastes. These are detected by the cilia of receptor cells in the taste buds, and are conducted by Cranial Nerve (CN)7 from the anterior 2/3 of the tongue, and CN 9 from the posterior 1/3 of the tongue, while adjacent trigeminal receptors conduct properties of pressure and touch (texture), temperature and pain via CN5.

Taste and trigeminal sensations make their way to the brainstem, the Nuclei Tractus Solaris or NTS (taste) and the Trigeminal Nucleus (sensations). They then travel along the gustatory and somatosensory tracts, respectively, to the midbrain to meet up with the olfactory input in the Insula and Prefrontal Gyrus.

Flow Chart for Orthonasal Smell: > = directs to

Aroma molecular compounds > nasal mucosa receptors > cribriform plate > glomeruli in olfactory bulb (pre-frontal cortex) > cells generate action potentials > olfactory tract takes two routes:

1. The lateral olfactory stria fibers project to CNS and medial temporal lobe > uncus, also the piriform cortex, the primary olfactory cortex > to amygdaloid complex > hypocampal gyrus (route for memory/emotion/conscious recognition)
2. The medial olfactory stria projects to peri-olfactory area, the subcallosal gyrus > insula and orbitofrontal cortex (route related to rewards/value).

Flow Chart for Taste: > = directs to

Receptors in the oral cavity, within the tastebuds and mucosal surfaces of the oropharynx, pharynx, epiglottis and esophagus are supplied by Cranial Nerves 7, 9, 10 and 12, with salivary secretion supplied by the motor branch of CN 7. Trigeminal sensations—pressure, touch, pain, and temperature, are conducted by CN 5.

1. Taste from the anterior 2/3 of the tongue conducts from the chorda tympani branch of CN 7 (Facial Nerve) >geniculate ganglion>

AND

2. Cranial Nerve 9 (glossopharyngeal) carries taste from the posterior 1/3 of the tongue >petrosal ganglion>
3. Cranial Nerve 10 (vagus) > pharynx/epiglottis>nodose ganglion>

All three > nucleus tractus solitarius (NTS) in the medulla >
then ascend via the pons >ventroposterior medial nucleus of the thalamus>through the internal capsule> to several areas, including:

hypocampus>	Insula (primary gustatory cortex)
hypothalamus>	Insula
amygdala>	Insula

Flow Chart for Somatosensory or Trigeminal > = directs to

Sensations >the lingual nerve branch of Cranial Nerve 5 > the trigeminal ganglion > trigeminal spinal nucleus caudalis in the medulla > trigeminal lemniscus (trigeminothalamic tract) which decussate to contralateral >VPM nucleus in thalamus >somatosensory cortex > Insula

ALL ROADS LEAD TO THE INSULA!

As you can see, when combined with the taste in foods or in smells that are food-associated, smell meets taste in the insula or insulary cortex. The insula is a para-limbic structure within the lateral sulcus. The insula's role is multi-sensory, affective, and cognitive processing involved with olfaction, and it communicates with olfactory, gustatory and other sensory association areas.

Gogolla (2017) described the insula as an anatomical "integration hub" for sensory processing and representation, feelings, emotions, autonomic and motor control, risk prediction, decision-making, bodily and self-awareness, and complex social functions, such as empathy.

WHERE FLAVOR IS CREATED

According to Veldhuizen et al. (2010), the insula receives input from many other parts of the brain, including those areas involving emotion and memory, but also from motor and other sensory pathways, and it is likely where the trigeminal components of flavor, such as temperature, touch, pressure and pain converge with smell and basic taste. The integrative properties of the insula appear to make it the best candidate for the center of flavor creation. In addition, learning takes place in the insula. The components of flavor lay down connections there and get reinforced through experience. So the insula appears to be the place where sensory training strikes gold!

WHY IS THIS IMPORTANT?

Understanding that the sensations of smell, taste, movement and position, temperature, light touch, pressure, and pain are directed through separate pathways yet meet up and integrate enables us to think about compensatory mechanisms, to find alternative ways to get sensory information to the brain, and in particular, to the insula.

Research in dysphagia studies, beginning with the work of the late Jerilyn Logemann in the 90s, has looked at bolus formation and latencies in transit time using various trigeminal effects. Thickening liquids, among the earliest efforts is most familiar, but later studies included temperature (cold), and flavor enhancers (sweet, sour). Among the most successful in affecting the mechanical aspects of mastication and swallow are the trigeminal effects of sour (Pauloski, 2016) and carbonation (Bulow, 2003; Michou 2012). Sour is a basic flavor but it's astringency is somatosensory. The bubbly aspect of carbonation is clearly a trigeminal component of flavor perception.

Beyond motor reactivity, we need to explore more of the trigeminal sensations, including burn (as in spicy), and textures, such as sticky, gummy, smooth, crunchy, slippery, creamy, and so on, that go beyond the familiar IDDSI dietary descriptions. Early gustatory memories no doubt encode these somato-sensations with taste as flavor perception. As such, they can help us form new neural connections for relearning by drawing on encoded memory. We should also try to evoke emotional memory as it may assist us in relearning flavor perception.

A key word is *compensatory*, because the information that will be relearned may actually be *alternatively* learned. Memory is not the same as real time. And aroma and flavor recreated are not the same as those first created by intact senses. We may recover or only learn a new version of those smell, taste and flavor perceptions. A new normal, if you will. Whether these new realities are entirely satisfactory to a patient is not for us to say.

Therefore, we can work with trigeminal stimuli and/or memories of odors, tastes and flavors to recover the old way of perceiving, or relearn a new version of reality. Or we can use these stimuli to provide entirely compensatory experiences. Let me give you an example of these two mechanisms.

1. Relearning. In the case of hyposmia, for example, with diminished smell acuity in the present, it's possible that a person can barely smell a lemon. Perhaps you can taste sour and sweet, however. And you have the puckering sensation of a sour lemon. You also have a sharp memory of the citrusy smell from a time you squeezed lemon into your tea or drank lemonade in the summer. Those sensations and perceptions, particularly ones from your childhood, may be attached to vivid and powerful memories. We can fill in the weak flavor experiences of the present with memories from the past. Through repeated stimulation, using present sensations fortified by memory, new nerve connections in the brain can possibly be established.
2. Compensatory. If a patient is discouraged about eating when favorite flavors cannot be experienced, or when flavors are unpleasantly distorted in the case

of parosmia or dysgeusia, we can enliven mealtime experiences by using compensatory strategies. We can chose foods, such as the ones suggested from the *Flavor Element Variables (FEVs)*, that permit the patient to focus on sensations and textures. Enjoy refreshing coolness, comforting warmth, spicy heat, crunchiness, smoothness or creaminess, even if they can't taste much of anything. When someone is parosmic, they may need to select foods that are cold and bland to suppress the volatile aromatics. If unpleasant flavors remain to any degree, the patient can boost potent somatosensory effects to distract themselves. Alternatively, they can replace unpleasant or bland flavors with those which won't offend or may even be exciting.

ACKNOWLEDGEMENTS

How did you spend the pandemic? I wrote this book, thanks to the inspiration of Catherine Lewis and support of Ritual Communications. I'm grateful to everyone who kept us safe and allowed us to reach this day, uninfected and alive to tell the tale. That includes all those I'll never get to thank personally, rarely ever thought about before 2020, yet who punched above their weight enabling us to keep our lives running. Obviously, I owe a debt of gratitude to an international community of epidemiologists, medical scientists, and olfactory investigators who have shared data that has informed my understanding, as well as kept me up nights. And to Pfizer, thanks for all the shots in the arm.

I can never thank my husband, N. J. Peluso, enough for doing his part, which included enduring my nearly incessant instructions on how to conduct our lives safely. His sound financial management made all that I have written here possible. On May 1, 2022, we lost our beloved canine daughter, Rhonda. She was approximately 20 years old. The love of our lives, she kept us company through the darkest of days. She will live forever in our hearts.

REFERENCES

de Araujo, I., Simon, S.(2009). The gustatory cortex and multisensory integration. *Int J Obes* 33, S34–S43._ https://doi.org/10.1038/ijo.2009.70

Aftel, M. (2008). *Essence and Alchemy: A Natural History of Perfume.* Gibbs Smith.

Altundag, A., Cayonu, M., Kayabasoglu, G., Salihoglu,M., Tekeli, H., Saglam, O., & Hummel, T, (2015). Modi!ed olfactory training in patients with post-infectious olfactory loss. *The Laryngoscope,* 125(8),1763–1766. https://doi.org/10.1002/lary.25245.

Altundag, A., Yilmaz, E., Kesimli, Caner, M. (2022). Modified Olfactory Training Is an Effective Treatment for COVID-19 Induced Parosmia. *The Laryngoscope.* 11:10.1002/lary.30101. https://doi:10.1002/lary.30101 [Epub ahead of print] PMCID:PMC9088368/ PMID35257391. Accessed online at ncbi.nlm.nih.gov

Antonelli, M., Pujal, J. C., Spector, T. D., Ourselin, S. &Steves, C. J. (2022) Risk of long COVID associated with delta versus omicron variants of SARS-CoV-2. *The Lancet.*399;10343, 263-2264. DOI: https://doi.org/10.1016/S0140-6736(22)00941-2.

Asimov, E. (2020, May 28). "Rediscovering Wine After Covid-19." The New York Times.

Ballering, A. V. , Van Zon, S. K. R., Hartman, T. C., Rosmalen, J. G. M. (2022) Persistence of somatic symptoms after COVID-19 in the Netherlands: an observational cohort study. *The Lancet*, August 6;400;10350;452-461. doi:https://doi.org/10.1016/S0140-67362201

Banks, S. J., Sreenivasan, K. R., Weintraub, D.M., Baldock, D., Noback, M., Pierce, M.E., Frasnelli, J., James, J. , Beall, E., Zhuang, X., Cordes, D. Leger, G. C.(2016) Structural and Functional MRI Differences in Master Sommeliers: A Pilot Study on Expertis in the Brain. *Front Human Neurosci.* ug 22;10:414. doi:103389/fnhum.2016.00414 PMD:27597821; PMCID:PMC4992723.

Barwich, A. S., (2020) *Smellosophy: what the nose tells the mind*, Harvard University Press.

Bitter, T., Gudziol, H., Burmeister, H.P., Mentzel, H.J., Guntinas-Lichius. O., & Gaser, C.(2010). Anosmia leads to a loss of gray matter in cortical brain areas. *Chem Senses.* 35(5):407-15. doi: 10.1093/chemse/bjq028. Epub 2010 Mar 15. PMID: 20231262.

Bitter, T., Brüderle, J,, Gudziol, H., Burmeister, H.P., Gaser, C. Guntinas-Lichius, O.(2010) Gray and white matter reduction in hyposmic subjects—A voxel-based morphometry study. *Brain Res.* Aug 6;1347:42-7. doi: 10.1016/j.brainres.2010.06.003. Epub 2010 Jun 8. PMID: 20553879.

Boscolo-Rizzo, P, Fabria, C., Polesel, J., Emanuelli, E., Tirelli, G., Spinato, G., Hopkins, C. (2022) Two-Year Prevalence and Recovery Rate of Altered Sense of Smell or Taste in Patients with Mildly Symptomatic COVID-19. *JAMA Otolaryngology-Head & Neck Surgery.* Published online August 4; doi10.1001/jamao-to.2022.1983.

Bosker, B., (2017). *Cork Dork: A Wine-Fueled Adventure Among The Obsessive Sommeliers, Big Bottle Hunters, and Rogue Scientist Who Taught Me to Live for Taste.* Penguin Books.

Boesveldt, S., Postma, E. M. & Duffy, V. B. (2017). Anosmia —A Clinical Review. *Chemical Senses.* Oxford University Press. September;42(7);607. Accessed online: ncbu.nlm.nih.gov

Brämerson, A., Johansson, L., Ek, L., Nordin, S., & Bende M. (2004). Prevalence of olfactory dysfunction: the skövde population-based study. *The Laryngoscope.* Apr;114(4): 733-7. https://doi:10.1097/00005537-200404000-00026. PMID:11064632.

Bull-Otterson L, Baca S, Saydah S, et al. (2022).Post–COVID Conditions Among Adult COVID-19 Survivors Aged 18–64 and ≥65 Years — United States, March 2020–November 2021. *MMWR Morb Mortal Wkly Rep.* 2022;71:713–717. DOI: http://dx.doi.org/10.15585/mmwr.mm7121e1

Bulow, M., Olsson, R., Ekberb, O. (2003). Videographic analysis of how carbonated thin liquids and thickened liquids affect the physiology of swallowing in subjects with aspiration on thin liquids. *Acta Radiol.* 44:366-372.

Cameron, E. L. (2014) Pregnancy and olfaction: a review. Fronteirs in psychology, 5,67. https://doi.org/10.3389/fpsyg.2014.00067

Carreira L, Midori Castelo, P., Simões, C., Capela e Silva, F., Viegas, C., Lamy, E. (2020). Changes in Salivary Proteome in Response to Bread Odour. *Nutrients.* 12(4):1002. https://doi.org/10.3390/nu12041002

Damm, M., Pikart, L.K., Reimann, H., Burkert, S., Goktas, O., Haxel, B., Frey, S., Charalampakis, I., Beule, A., Rener, B., Hummel,T., Huttenbrink, K.B. (2014) Olfactory training is helpful in post-infectious olfactory loss: a randomized, controlled, multi-center study. *The Laryngoscope* 124(4), pp826-831. Doi: 10.1002/lary.24340

Di Stadio, A., D'Ascanio, L., Vaira, L. A., Cantone, E., De Luca, P., Cingolani, C., Motta, G., De Riu, G., Vitelli, F., Spriano, G., De Vincentis, M., Camaioni, A., LaMantia, I., Ferreli, F., & Brenner, M. J., (2022). Ultramicronized Palmitoylethanolaimide and Luteolin Supplement Combined with Olfactory Training to Treat Post-COVID-19 Olfactory Impairment: A Multi-Center Double-Blinded Randomized Placebo-Controlled Clinical Trial. *Current neuropharmacology*, 10.2174/1570159X20666220420113513. Advance online publication. https://doi.org/10.2174/1570159X20666220420113513

Dong, J., Pinto, J. M., & Chen, H. (2017). The Prevalence of Anosmia and Associated Factors Among US Black and White Older Adults. *The Journal of Gerontology Series A: Biological Science and Medical Sciences.* J.Geronotol A. Biol Sci. Aug:72(8) 1080-1086. DOI:10:1093/GERONA/GLX081 Accessed at ncbi.nlm.nih.gov.

Douaud, G., Lee, S., Alfaro-Almagro, F., Arthofer, C., Wang,C., Lange, F., Andersson, J. L. R., Griffanti, L., Duff, E., Jbabdi, S., Taschler, B., Winkler, A., Nichols, T. E., Collins, R. Matthews, P. M., Allen, N., Miller, K.L., & Smith. S. M. (2021). Brain imaging before and after COVID-19 in UK Biobank. *MedRxiv* 06.11.21258690; doi: https://doi.org/10.1101/2021.06.11.21258690

Eliezer, M., Hamel, A., Houdart, E., Herman, P., Housset, J., Jourdaine, C., Eloit, C., Verillaud, B., Hautefort, C. (2020). Loss of smell in patients with COVID-19: MRI data reveal a transient edema of the olfactory clefts. *Neurology,* 95 (23) e3145-e3152. doi: 10.1212/WNL.0000000000010806

European Center for Disease Control, an agency of European Union. https://www.ecdc.europa.eu/en/covid-19/latest-evidence/clinical

Filiz, G., Poupon, D., Banks, S., Fernandez, P., & Frasnelli, J. (2022)Olfactory bulb volume and cortical thickness evolve during sommelier training. *Human Brain Mapping.* 43; 8.; 2621-2633. First published: 26 February 2022. https://doi.org/10.1002/hbm.25809

Frasnelli, J., Lundstrom, J. N., Boyle, J. A., Diordjievic, J., Zatorre, R. J., & Jones-Gotman, M. (2010). Neuroanatomical Correlates of Olfactory Performance. *Experimental Brain Research.* 201, 1-11.

Gilbert, A, (2014). *What the Nose Knows: The Science of Scent in Every Day Life*, Synesthetics, Inc.

Gogolla, N. (2017). The Insular Cortex. *Current Biology Magazine* 27, R573-R591, Elsevier Ltd.

Gupta, S., Lee, J. J., Perrin, A., Khan, A., Smith, H. J., Farrell, N., Kallogieri, D., Piccirillo, J.F. (2022) Efficacy and safety of saline nasal irrigation plus Theophylline for treatment of COVID-19-related olfactory dysfunction: the SCENT2 Phase2 randomized clinical trial. *JAMA Otolaryngol Head and Neck Surg.* 148(9) 830-837. doi:10.1001/jamaoto.2022.1573

Hoffman, H. J, Rawal, S., Li , C.M., & Duffy, V. B. *(2016).* New chemosensory component in the U.S. National Health and Nutrition Examination Survey (NHANES): first-year results for measured olfactory dysfunction. *Rev Endocr Metab Disord. 17:221–240.*

Holmes, B. (2017). *Flavor: The Science of Our Most Neglected Sense*, W. W. Norton & Company, Inc.

Hopkins, C., & Kelly, C. (2021) Prevalence and persistence of smell and taste dysfunction in COVID-19; how should dental practices apply diagnostic criteria? *BDJ In Practice. 34;22-23.* DOI: https://doi.org/10.1038/s41404-02100652-4

Hopkins, C., Kelley, C. E. (2022). AbScent online presentation March 29.

Hummel, T, Sekinger, B., Wolf, S. R., Pauli, E., & Kobal, G. (2020). 'Sniffin' Sticks': Olfactory Performance Assessed by the Combined Testing of Odor Identification, Odor Discrimination and Olfactory Threshold, https://acacemic.oup.com/chemse/article/221/39/383479 by guest on 09 September.

Ibekwe, T. S., Fasunla, A. J., & Orimadegun, A. E. (2020). Systematic Review and Meta-analysis of Smell and Taste Disorders in COVID-19. *OTO* open, 4(3), 2473974X20957975. https://doi.org/10.1177/2473974X20957975

Jiramongkolchai, P., Jones, M., Peterson, A., Lee, J.J., Liebendorfer, A., Klatt-Cromwell, C. N., Schneider, J. S., Drescher, A. J., Ogden, M.A., Brunworth, J. D., Kallogjeri, D., Kukuljan, S, Peelle, J. E., Piccirillo, J. F. (2021). Association of Olfactory Training with Neural Connectivity in Adults With Postviral Olfactory Dysfunction. *JAMA Otolaryngology Head & Neck Surgery.* Published online 18, March. doi:10.1001/jamaoto.2021.0086

Klein, J. (2017, May 11) . "Humans Have a Poor Sense of Smell? It's just a Myth," The New York Times.

Klein, J., Wood, J., Jaycox, J., Lu, P., Dhodapkar, R. M., Gehlhausen, J. R., Tabachnikova, A., Tabacof, L., Malik, A. M., Kamath, K., Greene, K., Monteiro, K. V. S., Peña-Hernandez, M. , Mao, T., Bhattacharjee, B.,Takahashi, T., Lucas, C., Silva, J., Mccarthy, D., Breyman, E., Tosto-Mancuso, J., Dai, Y., Perotti, E., Akduman, K., Tzeng, T. J., Xu, L., Yildirim, I., Krumholz, H. M., Shon, J., Medzhitov, R., Omer, S. B., van Dijk, D., M. Ring, A. M., Putrino, D., Iwasaki, A. (2022). Distinguishing features of Long COVID identified through immune profiling. *MedRxiv Pre-print Server.* 9 August 2022. https://doi.org/10.1101/2022.08.09.22278592

Kollndorfer, K., Fischmeister, F., Kowalczyk, K., Hoche, E., Mueller, C. A., Trattnig, S., & Schopf, V. (2015). Olfactory training induces changes in regional functional connectivity in patients with long-term smell loss. *NeuroImage: Clinical,*9; 401-410. https://doi.org/10.1016/j.nicl.2015.09.004

Langdon, C., Lehrer, E., Berenguer, J., Laxe, S., Alobid, I., Quintó, L., Mariño-Sánchez, F., Bernabeu, M., Marin, C., & Mullol, J. (2018). Olfactory Training in Post-Traumatic Smell Impairment: Mild Improvement in Threshold Performances: Results from a Randomized Controlled Trial. *Journal of neurotrauma,* 35(22), 2641–2652. https://doi.org/10.1089/neu.2017.5230

Liu, G., Zong, G., Doty, R. L., & Sun, Q. (2016). Prevalence and risk factors of taste and smell impairment in a nationwide representative sample of the US population : a cross- sectional study. *BMJOPEN* 2016;6:e013246. dpi:10.1136/bmjopen-2016-013246

Liu, D. T., Sabha, M., Damm, M., Philpott, C., Oleszkiewiz, A., Hanner, A., & Hummel, T. (2020). Parosmia is Associated with Relevant Olfactory Recovery After Olfactory Training. *The Larynoscope.* 131; 3, 618-623, 19 November. https://doi.org/10.1002/lary.29277

Malik, B., Elkaddi, N., Jumanah, T., Spielman, A., & Ozdener, M. H. (2019) Mammalian Taste Cells Express Functional Olfactory Receptors. *Chemical Senses.* May, 44(5):289-301. Published online 2019 April 23. DOI:10.1093/chemse/bjz019.

Malaty, J., & Malaty, I. A. (2013). Smell and taste disorders in primary care. *American family physicia*n, 88(12), 852–859.

Mc Gann, J. (2017). Poor human olfaction is a 19th-century myth. *Science.* 356, 597 12 May. DOI: 10.1126/science.aam7263

Mc Gee, H. (2020). *Nose Dive: A Field Guide to the World's Smells*, Penguin Press.

Mennella, J. A., Jagnow, C. P., & Beauchamp, G. K. (2001). Prenatal and postnatal flavor learning by human infants. *Pediatrics*, 107(6), E88. https://doi.org/10.1542/peds.107.6.e88

Michou, E., Mastan, A., Ahmed, S., Mistry, S., & Hamdy, S. (2012). Examining the Role of Carbonation and Temperature on Water Swallowing Performance: A Swallow Reaction-Time Study. *Chemical Senses* 37:790-807.
doi:10.1093/chemse/bjs061 July25, 2012, accessed through Researchgate.net.

Morquecho-Campos, P., Bikkers, F., Nazmi, K., Graaf, K. de., Laine, M. L., & Boesveldt, S. (2020). A stepwise approach investigating salivary responses upon multisensory food cues. *Physiology & Behavior.* November, Vol 226, 1. doi10.1016/j.physbeh.2020.113116.

O'Byrne, L., Webster, K .E, MacKeith, S, Philpott C, Hopkins, & C, Burton, M.J. (2022). Interventions for the treatment of persistent post-viral olfactory dysfunction. *Cochrane Database of Systematic Reviews.* 2022, Issue 2. Art. No.: CD014912. doi: 10.1002/14651858.CD014912.

Pellegrino, R., Mainland, J. D., Kelly, C. E., Parker, J. K., & Hummel,T. (2021). Prevalence and Correlates of Parosmia and Phantosmia among Smell Disorders. Pre-published doi: https://doi.org/10.1101/2021.07.02.21259925

Pauloski, B.R, & Nasir S.M. (2016). Orosensory contributions to dysphagia: a link between perception of sweet and sour taste and pharyngeal delay time. *Physiol Rep.* 4(11):e12752.

Poupon, D., Fernandez, P., & Frasnelli, J. (2019). Sommelier students display superior abilities to identify but not to detect or discriminate odors early in their training. *Chemosensory Perception.* 12, 106– 114. https://doi.org/10.1007/s12078-019-09256

Putrino, David. Interviews and speeches on Youtube.com

Rabin, R. C. (2020, 22 March). "Lost Sense of Smell May Be Peculiar Clue to Coronavirus Infection." The New York Times.

Schaal, B., Marlier, L., & Soussignan, R. (2000). Human foetuses learn odours from their pregnant mother's diet. *Chemical senses*, 25(6), 729-737. https://doi.org/10.1093/chemse/25.6.729

Shepherd, G.M. (2004). The human sense of smell: are we better than we think? *PLoS Biol.* May;2(5):E146. doi: 10.1371/journal.pbio.0020146. Epub 2004 May 11. PMID: 15138509; PMCID: PMC406401.

Shepherd, G. M. (2012) *Neurogastronomy: How the Brain Creates Flavor and Why It Matters.* Columbia University Press.

Stuckey, B. (2012) *Taste: Surprising Stores and Science about Why Food Tastes Good,* Atria Books.

Topol, E. (2022) Some Light on Long Covid: A cluster of new data. Ground Truths (newsletter) August 11.

Trimmera, C., Keller, A., Murphy, N. R., Snyder, L. L., Willerc, M. H., Nagaid, E. N., Katsanisc, L. B., Vosshallb, F, Matsunamid, H., & Mainlanda,J. D. (2019). Genetic Variation Across The Human Olfactory Receptor Repertoire Alters Odor Perception. *PNAS*, May 7; pnas.org/cgi/doi/10.107/pnas.1804106115

Vergara, J., Skoretz, S., Brodsky, M. B., Miles, A., Long,ore, S. E., Wallace, S., Seedat, J., Starmer, H. M., Bolton, L., Clave´, P., Freitas, S.V., Bogaardt, H., Matsuo, K., Madeira de Souza, C., & Mourão, L. F. (2020). Assessment, Diagnosis, and Treatment of Dysphagia in Patients Infected With SARS-CoV-2: A Review of the Literature and International Guidelines. *American Journal of Speech-Language Pathology, 29; Novemeber, 2242-2253.* https://doi.org/10.1044/2020_AJSLP-20-00163

Vergara J., Lirani-Silva, C., Brodsky, M.B., Miles, A., Clave´, P., Nascimiento, W. & Mourão, L. F. (2021) . Potential Influence of Olfactory, Gustatory, and Pharyngolaryngeal Sensory Dysfunctions on Swallowing Physiology in COVID-19. *Otolaryngology–Head and Neck Surgery, 164(6) 1134-1135.* doi:10.1177/0194599820972680

Veldhuizen, M. G., Nachtigal, D., Teulings, L., Gitelman, D. R., & Small, D. M. (2010). The Insular Taste CortexContributes To Odor Quality Coding. *Frontiers in Human Neuroscience,* July 21. Doi: 10.3389/fnhum.2010.000058

Yang, J., & Pinto, J.M. (2016) The Epidemiology of Olfactory Disorders. *Curr. Otorhinolaryngol Rep,* May;4(2):130-141. doi: 10.1007/s40136-016-0120-6. Epub 2016 Apr 7. PMID: 30613439; PMCID: PMC6317880.

World Health Organization, https://covid19.who.int

Zang, Y., Hahner, A., Negolas, S., Lakner, T. & Hummel, T. (2020). Apparently Minor Head Trauma Can Lead to Anosmia: A Case Report. *Journal for Oto-Rhino-Layrngology, Head and Neck Surgery,* published online Novemeber 11,2020. https://doi.org/10.1159/000511442

RESOURCES

STANDARDIZED TESTS

Smell and taste clinics and ENT specialists can use scientifically designed and standardized assessments for olfactory and gustatory impairments. However, many tests take time and may not allow for the time constraints experienced by many medical practitioners. Therefore, 1-minute and abbreviated tests are also listed below.

It is important to consider cultural differences when testing and many of these tests have controlled for them. The most recognized American tests include ones produced by Sensonics International (sensonics.com).

SMELL TESTS

QUICK OFFICE TESTS

1-minute office tests recommended to physicians

(Malaty & Malaty, 2013)

- Quick Smell Identification Test: Q-SIT/3-item, tear off-disposable
- Quick Sticks, Q-Sticks (subset of Sniffin Sticks)/3-item

The UPSIT— The University of Pennsylvania Smell Identification Test (American) is a 40-item scratch and sniff test that is considered the most accurate. Based on the work of Richard Doty, it is produced by Sensonics International. The UPSIT differentiates degree of smell loss and the ability to identify or discriminate odors. It is available in over 30 languages.

The B-SIT—The Brief Smell Identification Test is a 12-item test with a scratch and sniff format of odors that reportedly works across cultures. The Modified Brief Smell Identification Test identifies intensity, pleasantness and familiarity of odors. Available in Spanish and English.

The PST—The Pocket Smell Test is a 3-odor multiple choice, screening test. The 4-item NHANES Pocket Smell Test versions A and B were the basis of the National Health and Nutrition Examination Survey. Both PST versions are preliminary screenings meant to be followed up by more in-depth B-SIT or UPSIT in the event that a patient fails any items.

The ODMT- The Odor Discrimination Memory Test is a 12-item, non-verbal screening measure.

The Snap & Sniff Odor Discrimination Test composed of 20 scented wands. The test subject is required to choose which wand smells different. This is a costly test.

There are approximately 30 validated tests of some 200 that have been developed worldwide. The following two are well known and in in wide use.

The SST—The Sniffin' Sticks Test (Germany) is based on the work of Dr. Thomas Hummel of Dresden and is used widely in Central Europe. The SST has also proven valid for use in Spain. It presents 16 odorants in felt tip type pens. Hummel was also involved in the development of The Retronasal Smell Test which uses 20 odors presented as tasting powders applied to the tongue.

The SOIT—The Scandinavian Odor Identification Test (Sweden)

The SOIT tests for identification, discrimination and intensity (threshold) for 16 flask-presented scents, including 3 that stimulate the trigeminal nerve.

TASTE TESTS

- The WETT—Waterless Empirical Taste Test provides 50 taste strips of each stimulus: Sweet, Sour, Salty, Bitter, Umami (savory) and No-taste (control). Made by Sensonics (USA).
- The WETT-SA-53-The Self-Administered Waterless Empirical Taste Test is a 53-item version of The WETT.
- The B-WETT-SA-27- The Brief Self-Administered Waterless Empirical Taste Test is a 27- taste stimuli version of the WETT.
- The Retronasal Smell Test by Hummel (Germany) as previously mentioned (see Smell Tests).

ORGANIZATIONS

American Speech-Language-Hearing Association (ASHA) asha.org

monell.org

abscent.org

thefifthsense.org

thestana.org

patientresearchcovid19.com

Patient Led Research Collaborative organized by a group of Long COVID patients.

Long Covid Families: longcovidfamiies.org support and resources for families and children

@apresJ20 on Twitter (French)
ApresJ20-Association Covid Long France support group

@itsbodypolitic on Twitter

stasis.life (https://www.stasis.life)
for breathing and stress reduction
A video and coaching resource of breath techniques to improve physical and mental health. Helpful for those recovering from Covid, acute respiratory infections, allergies and asthma, dysautonomia, stress, fatigue and other issues.

International Dysphagia Diet Standardization Initiative (iddsi.org)
The IDDSI's mission is to achieve standardization in the description of food textures used in medical, rehabilitative and therapeutic settings so to enable professionals, patients and caregivers to communicate with precision.

ecdc.europa.eu
European Center for Disease Control (European Union)

cdc.gov Center for Disease Control (USA)

POST ACUTE COVID SYNDROME (LONG COVID) TREATMENT

The Mount Sinai Hospital Post Acute Covid Clinic, New York, NY

The Mount Sinai School of Medicine Rehabilitation Innovation Program Director: David Putrino, PhD.

A ground-breaking 100-day physical therapy program, aimed at patients suffering debilitating, dysautonomia-like symptoms, such as, fatigue, brain fog, and disorders of the gastrointestinal, cardio-vascular and respiratory systems.

DIETARY RESOURCES FOR ANOSMIA

BOOKS

Taste & Flavour
by Ryan Riley & Kimberly Duke, Bloomsbury Publishing, First Edition (2005)
https://lifekitchen.co.uk

WEBSITES

Miranda's Anosmic Kitchen
myanosmickitchen.com

CHEWING AND SWALLOWING DISABILITIES (DYSPHAGIA)

Savorease Therapeutic Foods

savorease.com

Designed by a dentist with a culinary background, these tasty wafers can be used to practice biting and chewing, strengthening oral muscles while providing nutritious snacks. The wafers quickly melt down to puree consistency for safe swallowing by those on a puree diet.

Dysphagia Research Society dysphagiaresearch.org

National Foundation of Swallowing Disorders
https://swallowingdisorderfoundation.com

BREATHING REHABILITATION DEVICES/EXPIRATORY MUSCLE STRENGTH TRAINING (EMST)

The Breather ® : pnmedical.com

EMST150 ® : emst150.com

Expand-a Lung ® :expand-a-lung.com

SMELL AND TASTE CLINICS

Research is emerging from university-affiliated hospitals in most major cities across the world at the time of this writing. If you're looking for treatment, start with the otolaryngology departments. The following is a partial list of clinics specializing in smell and taste disorders.

UNITED STATES OF AMERICA

CALIFORNIA

Nasal Dysfunction Clinic at UCSD
University of California, San Diego, Medical Center
200 W. Arbor Drive
San Diego, CA 92103-8654

Stanford Otolaryngology – Head & Neck Surgery
801 Welch Road
Palo Alto, CA 94304 Phone: 650-723-5281

COLORADO

Chemosensory Perception Lab, (UCSD)
Colorado at Rocky Mountain Smell and Taste Center
University of Colorado Health Science Center
4200 E. Ninth Avenue
Denver, CO 80262

CONNECTICUT

Connecticut Chemosensory Clinical Research Center
Taste and Smell Center at the University of Connecticut Health Center
263 Farmington Avenue
Farmington, CT 06030

WASHINGTON D.C.

Taste and Smell Clinic, Washington, DC
Taste and Smell Clinic
5125 MacArthur Blvd., Suite 20
Washington, D.C. 20016
E-mail: Doc@TasteandSmell.com
Phone Number: 202-364-4180 F
AX Number: 202-364-9727

MARYLAND

National Institute of Dental Research
National Institutes of Health
NIH Bldg. 10, Room 1N-114
Bethesda, MD 20892

Johns Hopkins Medical Center
(410) 955-5000

NEW YORK

Clinical Olfactory Research Center
State University of New York Health Science
Center at Syracuse College of Medicine
766 Irving Avenue Syracuse, NY 13210

Columbia/New York Presbyterian
Department of Otolaryngology
180 Fort Washington Ave.
7th Floor
New York, NY 10032
(212) 305-8555

ILLINOIS

Smell & Taste Treatment and Research Foundation, Ltd
233 East Erie Street, Suite 702
Chicago, Illinois 60611
(888) 381- 8040; (847) 274-2267

OHIO

University of Cincinnati Taste and Smell Center
University of Cincinnati College of Medicine
231 Bethesda Avenue
Cincinnati, OH 45267-0528
And:
Cincinnati Smell Lab

The Department of Otolaryngology, University of Cincinnati

PENNSYLVANIA

Smell and Taste Center at the Hospital of the University of Pennsylvania
Crystal Wylie, Patient Coordinator
Smell and Taste Center
Hospital of University of Pennsylvania
3400 Spruce Street, 5 Ravdin
Philadelphia, PA 19104-4283
Phone: (215) 662-2797 Fax: (215) 349-5266
Email Crystal.Wylie@uphs.upenn.edu

TENNESSEE

Vanderbilt University Medical Center/Bill Wilkerson Center
Smell and Taste Clinic/Dept. of Otolaryngology
1215 21st Ave. S., Floors 6-10
Nashville, TN 37232
(615)936-5000
Vanderbilt has additional locations

TEXAS

Taste & Smell Disorders Clinic
Seton Center Lakeway
1602 Lohmans Crossing
Austin, Texas 78734
off: 512 2617909
fax: 512 2611736

VIRGINIA

MCV Smell and Taste Clinic
Medical College of Virginia Richmond,
VA 23298-0551

UNITED KINGDOM

Clinics in the UK require referrals from General Practitioners
Check for regional branches of the Royal College of General Practitioners
Royal College of General Practitioners 30 Euston Square London NW1 2FB
Email: info@rcgp.org.uk
Tel : 020 3188 7400

Rhinology Clinics at Imperial College Hospitals
NHS Foundation Trust, Charing Cross Hospital
Fulham Palace Road, W6 8RF
Tel: 020 3311 1025

The Sinus Clinic at Royal Surrey County Hospital
Egerton Road, Guildford, GU2 7XX.
Tel: 01483 571122

Rhinology Clinic at Guys Hospital
London, SE1 9RT

Joint Nasal Clinic. Royal London Hospital
Whitechapel Rd,
Whitechapel, London E1 1FR

The Norfolk Smell & Taste Clinic
The Norfolk & Waveney ENT Service
Norwich Medical School
University of East Anglia

The Smell and Taste Clinic at James Paget Hospital
James Paget University Hospital,
Gorleston, Great Yarmouth, NR31 6LA.
Tel: 01493 452832

The Smell and Taste Clinic at Birmingham Queen Elizabeth Hospital
Queen Elizabeth Medical Centre
Birmingham B15 2TH
Tel: 0121 627 2000

Rhinology Clinic at Freeman Hospital
High Heaton, Newcastle, NE7 7DN.
Tel: 0191 2137635

Rhinology Service at Aintree Hospital,
Liverpool L9 7AL

SCOTLAND

Contact for lists of practitioners.

Queen Elizabeth University Hospital
1345 Govan Road, Govan,
Glasgow, G51 4TF
Main Switchboard:
0141 201 1100
Private hospitals in Glasgow: www.bmihealthcare.co.uk/ross-hall www.nuffieldhealth.com/glasgowhospital

University of Edinburgh
Otolaryngology Units
Royal Infirmary of Edinburgh and Western General
NHS Secretary: 0131 536 4453

Edinburgh ENT practice at the Spire Hospitals in Edinburgh
The Murrayfield Hospital
122 Corstorphine Road, Edinburgh, EH12 6UD
0131 3340363

The Spire Shawfair Park Hospital
10 Easter Shawfair, Edinburgh, EH22 1FE
0131 6545600

GERMANY

Smell and Taste Clinic
University of Dresden Medical School
Fetscherstrasse 74, 01307
Dresden, Germany
Tel: +49-351-458-4189

GREECE

Smell and Taste Clinic
Aristotle University, Papageorgiou Hospital
Efkarpia Ring Road,
Thessaloniki, Greece
Tel: 0030 2313323523

SPAIN

Check Otolaryngology Departments at university hospitals in the major cities, such as:
Rhinology Unit & Smell Clinic, ENT Department,
Hospital Clinic Barcelona, Barcelona, Catalonia, Spain.

SWEDEN

Department of Otorhinolaryngology
Karolinska University Hospital,
Huddinge, Stockholm, Sweden

CANADA

BRITISH COLUMBIA

St Paul's Sinus Centre
St Paul's Hospital Foundation
178 – 1081 Burrard Street, Vancouver, BC V6Z 1Y6
Tel: (Metro Vancouver): 604-682-8206
(BC toll free) 800-720-2983

Canadian Society of Otolaryngology http://www.entcanada.org lists the following:

University of British Columbia, VANCOUVER, BC
Gordon & Leslie Diamond Health Care Centre
4th Floor, 2775 Laurel St., DHCC VGH
Vancouver, BC V5Z 1M9
Tel: (604) 875-4664 / Fax: (604) 875-5018

BC Children's Hospital, K2-184
4480 Oak St.
Vancouver,
BC V6H 3V4
Tel: (604) 875-2345 ex 5191

NOVA SCOTIA

Dalhousie University, HALIFAX, NS
Dickson Building, Room 3052
5820 University Ave.
Halifax, NS B3H 1V8
Tel: (902) 473-5752/Fax: (902) 473-4016

QUEBEC

Université Laval, QUÉBEC, QC
Hôpital de l'Enfant-Jésus du CHU de Québec
1401, 18e Rue
Québec (Québec) G1J 1Z4
Lucie Aubin, Agente de secrétariat
Département d'ophtalmologie et d'oto-rhino-laryngologie – chirurgie cervico-faciale Tél: (418) 656-2131 poste 413010

Université de Sherbrooke, SHERBROOKE, QC
CHUS-Hotel Dieu, 580 Bowen sud
Sherbrooke, QC J1G 2E8
Tel: (819) 346-1110 ex 14901/ Fax: (819) 564-5449

McGill University, MONTREAL, QC
Department of Otolaryngology-Head and Neck Surgery
687 Pine Ave. West, Room E3-37
Montreal, PQ H3A 1A1
Tel: (514) 843-2820 / Fax: (514) 843-1403

McGill University Health Centre Glen Site, Royal Victoria Hospital
1001 Decaire Boul., #D05.5711
Montreal, QC H4A 3J1
RVH (514) 843-2820

Department of Otolaryngology – Head & Neck Surgery
McGill University, MUHC (Royal Victoria Hospital)
1001 boul. Decarie – D05.5641
Montreal, QC H4A 3J1
Tel: (514) 934-1934 ext.32820

Université de Montréal, MONTRÉAL, QC
Div of Otolaryngology-Head & Neck Surgery
5415 boul L'Assomption
1er etage, pav. J.A. DeSeve, porte JD 1107 Montreal, PQ H1T 2M4
Tel: (514) 252-3400 ex. 7267

ONTARIO

University of Ottawa, OTTAWA, ONTARIO
Department of Otolaryngology-Head and Neck Surgery
Ottawa Hospital, General Campus
501 Smyth Rd. Ottawa, ON K1H 8L6
Tel: (613) 737-8899; (613)722-7000
Alternate address: 263 – 737 Parkdale Ave. Ottawa, ON K1Y 1J8
Phone: (613) 798-5555 Ext. 13631 / Fax: (613) 761-4356

University of Toronto
Department of Otolaryngology-Head & Neck Surgery
C. David Nader Bldg.
120 – 6 Queen's Park Cres. W.
Toronto, ON M5S 3H2
Tel: (416) 946-8742 / Fax: (416) 946-8744

Mc Master University, HAMILTON, ONTARIO
Division of Otolaryngology – Head & Neck Surgery
Department of Surgery
St. Joseph's Healthcare
50 Charlton Ave. E., Room G819
Hamilton, ON L8N 4A6
Tel: (905) 522-1155 x35804; Fax: (905) 522-4644

Division of Otolaryngology-Head and Neck Surgery
4E12 – 1280 Main St. West
Hamilton, ON L8N 3Z5
Tel: (905) 521-2100 / Fax: (905) 521-8552

Western University, LONDON, ONTARIO
Department of Otolaryngology-Head and Neck Surgery
800 Commissioners Rd. E.,Room C3-100
London, ON N6A 5W9
Tel: (519) 685.8500 ex 55807

St. Joseph Health Care
268 Grosvenor St., B2-501
London, ON N6A 4V2
Tel: (519) 685-8500 ex 66320

MANITOBA

University of Manitoba, WINNIPEG, MB
HSC-GB421, 820 Sherbrook Street
Winnipeg, MB R3A 1R9
Tel: (204) 787-7773 / Fax: (204) 787-1727
Administrative Office: (204) 787-3349

ALBERTA

University of Calgary, CALGARY, AB
Division of Otolaryngology-Head & Neck Surgery
RRDTC – ENT Clinic RM 21304E, 1820 Richmond Rd. S.W.
Calgary, AB T2N 5C7
Tel: (403) 955-9059 / (403) 282-0054 / Fax: (403) 955-8779

University of Alberta, EDMONTON, AB
Division of Otolaryngology-Head and Neck Surgery
Department of Surgery
1E4.33 WMC, 8440 – 112 Street
Edmonton, AB T6G 2B7
Tel: (780) 407-3691 / Fax: (780) 407-2004

MEXICO

The ABC Hospital(American British Cowdray Medical Center) is located in Mexico City. Call them for referrals in other parts of Mexico.
Av. Carlos Graef Fernández 154,
Col. Santa Fe, Cuajimalpa,
05300, Cd. de México.
Tel. 55 1103 1600

Smell and Taste Clinic
Hospital ABC Campus Santa Fe, consultorio 154
Tel: 1664 7078;1664 7079
Email: gustoyolfayto@gmail.com

ABOUT THE AUTHOR

R. M. Peluso is an ASHA-certified Speech-Language Pathologist who writes under her married name, but has been in clinical practice for over 30 years using her maiden name. Much of her career involved working with dysphagia (swallowing disorders). R. M. began her tasting career in 2006, writing for the C-Spot®, the leading online premium chocolate review site. As a food writer, she has been a regular contributor to Cheese Connoisseur Magazine and Whisky Magazine (UK). She is the author of *Deep Tasting: A Chocolate Lover's Guide to Meditation* and *Deep Tasting: Chocolate and Whiskey. Recovery of Smell and Taste* is her third book.

INDEX

Printed in Great Britain
by Amazon

43888333R00129